# Mathematics for Dyslexics

## A Teaching Handbook

STEPHEN J. CHINN and J. RICHARD ASHCROFT

*Mark College, Somerset*

Consulting Editor in Dyslexia: Professor Margaret Snowling,
University of Newcastle upon Tyne

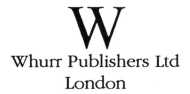

Whurr Publishers Ltd
London

© 1993 Whurr Publishers Ltd

First published 1993 by
Whurr Publishers Ltd
19b Compton Terrace, London N1 2UN, England

Reprinted 1993, 1994 (twice) and 1995

**British Library Cataloguing-in-Publication Data.**
A catalogue record for this book is available from the
British Library

ISBN 1-870332-74-1

Singular number 1-565932-50-1

Photoset by Edgerton Publishing Services, Huddersfield
Printed and bound in the UK by
Athenæum Press Ltd, Gateshead, Tyne & Wear

# Preface

Although there is a wide range of material available to help in teaching language to dyslexic children, there is very little available for teaching mathematics. This book offers practical advice gleaned from 20 years of classroom experience of teaching mathematics to dyslexic children.

We have learnt that there is no single answer for problems with teaching and learning. Each class we meet is a reminder that every child has individual needs, even if grouped around a basic common core of needs. To address these needs, we have developed a flexible approach, based on a knowledge of dyslexia and an understanding of the nature of mathematics.

We have collected, tested and organised the most effective ideas from many sources, including material for pupils ranging from low attainers through to those who will reach the highest levels. Subjects covered go back to first principles to act at the root of the problem.

The contents and structure of this book are such that they can be applied to class or individual teaching, for children from year 1 to year 13, and to dyslexic children or other children who are having difficulties with mathematics.

We would like to point out that we have tended to use the pronoun 'he' more often than 'she' in the text; this is because the ratio of dyslexic boys to dyslexic girls is 4:1, and so it seems more appropriate to use 'he'.

**Steve Chinn**
**Richard Ashcroft**
April 1993

# Dedications

For Emily, Jamie, Simon and Sarah (SJC), for Steve Marr and George Adie (JRA) and for all the dyslexic mathematicians who have taught us so much.

**Steve Chinn**
**Richard Ashcroft**

# Contents

## Chapter 12    162

## Decimals

## Chapter 13    181

## Percentages

## Chapter 14

## Introducing Other Topics

## Chapter 15    198

## The Teaching Programme at Mark College

# Chapter 1
# Dyslexia and Mathematics

## Introduction

When we moved from working in mainstream schools and began teaching in schools for dyslexic pupils, our initial expectation was that teaching mathematics would be much the same as before. At that time (1981) we could not find a source of guidance to confirm or contradict this expectation. We thought dyslexia meant difficulties with language, not mathematics. Experience would change this impression!

Over the last 12 years we have accumulated experience, tried out new ideas, researched, read what little material was available, studied in the USA, and have become convinced that difficulties in mathematics go hand in hand with difficulties in language and that a different teaching approach is needed. The first three chapters of this book look at some of the background to the development of these teaching methods and the remaining chapters describe the methods used.

## Definitions of Dyslexia

A brief survey of definitions of dyslexia (and learning disabilities, an American term) shows how difficulties with mathematics have been introduced alongside difficulties with language. Only 23 years ago MacDonald Critchley (1970) defined dyslexia as

> A disorder manifested by a difficulty in learning to read, despite conventional instruction, adequate intelligence and socio-cultural opportunity. It is dependent upon fundamental cognitive difficulties which are frequently of a constitutional character.

Mathematics was also absent in the definition provided in 1968 by the World Federation of Neurology.

In 1972 the Department of Education and Science for England and Wales did include number abilities in its definition of specific reading (*sic*)

1

difficulties. In the USA, the Interagency Conference (Kavanagh and Truss, 1988) defined learning disabilities to include 'significant difficulties in the acquisition of mathematical abilities' and, in the UK, Chasty (1989) defined specific learning difficulties as

> organising or learning difficulties, which restrict the student's competence in information processing, in fine motor skills and working memory, so causing limitations in some or all of the skills of speech, reading, spelling, writing, essay writing, numeracy and behaviour.

By 1992 Miles and Miles, in their book *Dyslexia and Mathematics*, wrote:

> The central theme of this book is that the difficulties experienced by dyslexics in mathematics are manifestations of the same limitations which also affect their reading and spelling.

## Resources

There is a paucity of research in this field, as noted by Austin (1982), Sharma (1986) and Miles and Miles (1992). The foremost publication on dyslexia in the USA, the *Annals of the Orton Dyslexia Society*, had not one paper on mathematics in the five years from 1986 to 1991. In the UK *Specific Learning Difficulties (Dyslexia): Challenges and Responses* (Pumphrey and Reason, 1991) again only makes passing reference to numeracy and mathematics.

There is, however, some reference material. Steeves (1979) looked at multisensory mathematics and other ideas to help teachers working with dyslexics. Steeves advocated the same teaching principles as Orton had suggested for language. Joffe (1983) provided an excellent overview of the relationship between dyslexia and mathematics. Within this relatively short paper, Joffe provides many observations which add to a clearer understanding of difficulties in mathematics, most notably that there is a weakness in the essential skill of generalising.

Sometimes the advice given is contradictory. Ashlock et al. (1983) in an otherwise useful book state that all children learn and come to understand an idea in basically the same way, whereas Bley and Thornton (1989) start their book with the sentence, 'Learning disabled children are unable to learn the way most children do'. (We consider the latter statement to be the correct one.)

*Dyslexia and Mathematics* (Miles and Miles, 1992) collects together a wealth of material, including a thorough review of the history of dyslexia and mathematics and a range of practical ideas for teachers. The journal, *Focus on Learning Problems in Mathematics* and the associated *Math Notebook* provide ongoing support.

# Dyscalculia

The problem of a specific mathematics difficulty, dyscalculia, needs some mention. The term suggests learning difficulties which are solely related to mathematics. The little research that exists suggests that the proportion of children in this category is small. In a study by G. Hitch (1991, private communication) of 1200 children aged 9 to 12, only 18 were identified as having specific mathematics difficulties. Sutherland (1988) states that on the basis of his study, few children have specific problems with number alone. Rather, Miles (in Miles and Miles, 1992) suggests that mathematical difficulties and language difficulties are likely to occur concurrently and we come to the same conclusion in the last part of this chapter. The work of Kosc, a pioneer in the field of dyscalculia, and a review of the literature on dyscalculia can be found in *Focus on Learning Difficulties in Mathematics* (Sharma, 1986).

# The Nature of Mathematics

In order to teach successfully, you need a knowledge of the pupil and a knowledge of the subject. To teach mathematics effectively you must have some understanding of the nature of mathematics and its progression beyond the immediate topics being taught. It is a subject which builds on previous knowledge as it extends knowledge. What can create significant problems are programmes which require mastery before progression because mastery, especially of rote learning tasks, is a transient stage for many dyslexics.

Numbers can be exciting, challenging tools (McLeish, 1991) or the cause of great anxiety (Buxton, 1981; Cope, 1988). Mathematics is a sequential subject, building on early skills and knowledge to take the student on to new skills and knowledge. It is a subject of organisation and patterns (Ashcroft and Chinn, 1992), of abstract ideas and concepts. Gaps in the early stages of understanding can only handicap the learner in later stages, in the speed of processing number problems if nothing else.

Mathematics has an interrelating/sequential/reflective structure. It is a subject where one learns the parts; the parts build on each other to make a whole; knowing the whole enables one to reflect with more understanding on the parts, which in turn strengthens the whole. Knowing the whole also enables one to understand the sequences and interactions of the parts and the way they support each other so that the getting there clarifies the stages of the journey. Teachers are (usually) in the fortunate position of being conversant with the subject and can bring to the work knowledge and experience beyond the topic they are teaching. The pupil is rarely in this position and thus is vulnerable to assumptions about his levels of knowledge and experience, often made unconsciously by the teacher.

It is important that the pupil develops a clear and diverse understanding of number at each stage, that he begins to see the interrelationships, patterns, generalisations and concepts clearly and without anxiety. To teach a child to attain this understanding of mathematics requires that you also need to understand mathematics and numbers. This is not to say that every teacher who teaches arithmetic needs a degree in mathematics, but it is to say that you need to understand where mathematics is going beyond the level at which you teach, so that what you teach is of benefit to the child at the time and helps, not hinders, him later on as his mathematics develops. You need to be mindful of what is coming after what you have taught, because the development of a concept starts long before it is addressed directly.

To illustrate this point consider the strategy advocated in this book for teaching the nine times table (see Chapter 6). The method uses previous information (the ten times table), estimation, refinement of estimation and patterns. Although a child may not need to realise that he is doing all these things when he learns how to work out $6 \times 9$, the processes are being used, concepts are being introduced and foundations are being laid.

Margaret Rawson said of teaching English to dyslexics 'Teach the language as it is to the child as he is'. Harry Chasty says 'If the child does not learn the way you teach, then you must teach the way he learns'. This advice is apposite for teaching mathematics. You need to understand the way each child learns as an individual, though individual learning can be frustrating in that a lesson which works superbly with one child may not work at all with another (see Chapter 2). This combined understanding of the child and all his strengths, weaknesses and potentials plus a knowledge of the nature, structure and skills of mathematics will help to make you an effective teacher.

## Factors which may contribute to learning difficulties in mathematics

Different children bring different combinations of strengths and weaknesses to mathematics. These will interact with the subject and the learning situation to create different levels of success and failure. Homan (1970) and Chinn (1991) have looked at deficits which may affect performance in mathematics. These deficits combine to form a large part of the picture of what the child brings to the problem. Each deficit may make a different contribution to the overall problem, ensuring an enormous range of variation among children, which is typical of dyslexia. A knowledge of the deficits provides a general background which you must have firmly fixed in your mind as you individualise your approach to each child or as you work with a group.

# Potential Areas of Difficulty in the Realm of Mathematics

### Directional confusion

Children may write numbers backwards, $\varepsilon$ for 3, or may be confused by the inconsistent 'starting points' of algorithms, e.g. addition, where the child starts at the right and works left:

$$362$$
$$+\,431$$

and worse, subtractions, where the child starts at the bottom right and has to remember to 'take' the lower number from the top number, 'borrow' from the left upper number and move left:

$$495$$
$$-236$$

or long division, where the child has to start at the left and move right and downwards while writing the answer at the top:

$$5\overline{)2655}$$

### Sequencing problems

It may be difficult for a child to count, especially using one-to-one correspondence. It is frequently difficult for a child to count backwards. Children may write 18 as 81 (which has some logic) or 26 as 62 (which doesn't) (Sharma, 1987). They may have difficulty remembering the sequence of steps to follow for long division. It may be difficult for a child to see a sequence (for example, $4^0\ 4^1\ 4^2\ 4^3$).

### Visual perceptual difficulties

The pupil may confuse +, ÷ and × (especially if written carelessly) or 6 and 9 or 3 and 5.

### Spatial awareness

Spatial awareness is needed for work such as place value or distinguishing between 2 and $z$ or three-dimensional geometry. In the classroom the pupil may lose his place on the page (or board) from which he is copying. He may not be able to relate two-dimensional drawings to the three-dimensional shape they represent.

## Short-term (working) memory

Poor short-term memory can create several areas of difficulty and has a strong influence on how a pupil processes numbers. Deficits in short-term memory combined with long-term memory deficits create major problems. For example, a child trying to add 47 and 78 mentally has to hold the sum in his memory, probably work out $7 + 8$ (poor memory for basic facts), remember 5, carry 1, remember that he has to add 4 and 7 (and the carried 1), work out $7 + 4 + 1$, recall the 5 and put them all together in the right sequence 125.

Short-term memory difficulties may even prevent a pupil from starting a problem; he may simply forget some or all of the teacher's instructions or, if his short-term memory is overloaded, he may be left with absolutely no clues as to where to start. The pupil may not be able to 'hold' the visual image of the sum he is trying to solve. He may not be able to hold the sum in visual or auditory memory while he searches for a necessary number fact. (Indeed the working out of that fact, say $9 + 6$ by counting on, may overload the memory and leave him not remembering the initial sum.)

## Long-term memory

Rote learning as a means of loading information into long-term memory is rarely effective with dyslexics (Pritchard et al., 1989), though teachers still persist in trying (McDougal, 1990). Dyslexics have significant difficulties learning basic facts such as times tables (Pritchard et al., 1989). This is particularly frustrating for parents who encourage the child to practise until he achieves mastery one day only to find that the child has forgotten again soon after.

Poor long-term memory may also handicap other areas of mathematics, such as recall of algorithms (methods) or formulae.

## The language of mathematics: difficulties in naming

Mathematics has its own language and symbols and this brings further problems for the dyslexic whose language skills may be weak. To complicate the issue further, the same symbol often has different names, e.g. + means add, more, plus, positive, and (Henderson, 1989).

## Word skills (Kibel, 1992; E. Miles, 1992)

A child needs to be able to read a problem with accuracy (and a certain amount of speed). The wording for mathematics problems tends to be precise and so needs accurate reading and interpretation. A child who misses key words or perhaps small words such as 'not' will be disadvantaged.

**Cognitive style** (see Chapter 2)

The child's cognitive style, the way he works out a problem, is significantly influenced by the factors above. It may not match the teacher's cognitive style. Some writers use the terms learning and teaching style, which often refer to classroom styles, for example, informal or formal, a management aspect. Although this is relevant in that a teacher whose style is predominantly verbal will disadvantage a child whose style is predominantly visual, we are referring here to the cognitive styles of teacher and learner.

This particular facet of mathematics learning and teaching was highlighted by Cockcroft (1982) who stated (§242):

> We are aware that there are some teachers who would wish us to indicate a definitive style for the teaching of mathematics, but we do not believe this is either desirable or possible.

and, later (§256)

> ...The now well established fact that those who are mathematically effective in daily life seldom make use 'in their heads' of the standard written methods which are taught in the classroom.

**Conceptual ability**

The child's ability to form concepts will be aided by the range and extent of the experiences he receives. 'Drill and practice' is often used to reinforce a new topic. A dyslexic student is typically slower and will often manage less practice for this reason alone. A child who continually fails in mathematics will also have a smaller variety of experiences and consequently will be less likely to be able to see patterns and to generalise and thus to form concepts. This has the effect of compounding his difficulties and retarding his progress.

**Anxiety and self-image**

Overlaying all the above areas of difficulty is the child's poor self-image and his mathematics anxiety (Buxton, 1981). This is a cumulative and cyclic problem – more failure, more anxiety, more failure, poorer self-image, more failure, etc.

# Summary

The definition of dyslexia has been expanded from a consideration of just language difficulties to include numeracy/arithmetic difficulties. There is now a greater awareness that difficulties in mathematics frequently occur concurrently with language difficulties.

Mathematics is a sequential subject, so if early difficulties are not addressed effectively then 'classroom-acquired' difficulties will be added to inherent difficulties and compound the child's failure. If the remediation is started at the right time but is too slow, or continues for too short a time, the extent of the child's problems will still be increasing for, while his peers progress, the dyslexic child will be marking time (or even regressing).

Thus it seems recognised that many dyslexics have difficulty in at least some aspects of mathematics, but this is not, necessarily, in all areas of mathematics. Indeed some dyslexics are gifted problem solvers, despite persisting difficulties in, for example, rote learning of basic facts. An inappropriate education may leave such a child floundering in early numeracy when he has the ability to leapfrog over these difficulties into more advanced aspects of mathematics. If the problem is not appropriately (and continuously) addressed, these learning difficulties may reduce the extent of the child's mathematical experiences, making it harder for him to develop concepts and to progress past the very basic levels of knowledge. The difficulty may create a cumulative effect beyond its original potential, if it is not addressed at an early stage (and thereafter).

As the teacher, you require both an understanding of the strengths and weaknesses which the child brings to each lesson and a knowledge of the structure and interrelating nature of mathematics. It is the successful interaction of these items of knowledge which helps to make an effective teacher.

# Chapter 2
# Cognitive Style in Mathematics

## Introduction

Cognitive style in mathematics refers to the way a person thinks through a problem. Its history can be dated back as far as Descartes (1638, cited in Krutetskii, 1976), who described two styles of problem-solver. The first solves problems by a succession of logical deductions, whilst the second uses intuition and immediate perceptions of connections and relationships. These two contrasting styles are described again in later literature. Boltevskii (1908, cited in Krutetskii, 1976) and Harvey (1982) labelled the two styles geometers and algebraists, where the algebraist links most closely to the logical, sequential thinker and the geometer to the intuitive style. Kovalev and Myshishchev (Krutetskii, 1976) used the term 'intuitive' to describe a person who is not conscious of every step in his thought processes but who perceives essential connections more clearly and quickly than his complementary stylist, the 'discursive' thinker.

Although Polya (1962) identified four styles of problem-solver, the four can readily be combined in pairs, reducing them to two distinct styles. Polya called the four styles groping, bright idea, algebra and generalisation. The first two describe intuitive thinkers and the last two describe sequential thinkers.

## Qualitative and Quantitative Style

More recently, Sharma (1986, 1989) identified and labelled two extreme styles (personalities) as quantitative and qualitative. The characteristics of the quantitative style are essentially sequential/logical and those of the qualitative are intuitive and holistic. Sharma also suggested that most personalities lie on a continuum between these two extremes. He uses the order in which the Rey Osterrieth Complex Figure is copied as one of the instruments to diagnose the preferred learning personality. This figure

9

(Figure 2.1) is detailed and Sharma looks to see if the detail takes precedent over the outline when the figure is reproduced.

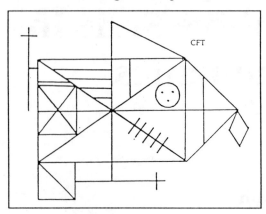

**Figure 2.1**    The Rey Osterrieth Complex Design Test

Sharma's qualitative learner approaches problems holistically and is good at spotting patterns. He uses an intuitive approach, tends not to show his working and does not like practice exercises. This contrasts with the quantitative learner who processes information sequentially, looking for formulae, methods and 'recipes'. This learner attempts to classify problems into types and to identify a suitable process to use in solving the problem.

It is worth noting that the intuitive style is not always viewed favourably. For example, Skemp (1971) considered it a hit-and-miss method, which is not always reproducible. Most people have experience of the teacher who says, 'I am not marking that mathematics until I can see some method written down'. (Whilst there are some very valid reasons for this to be a reasonable comment, it often indicates a lack of understanding of learning style.)

## The brain

Some writers have linked cognitive style to hemispheric specialisation. Kane and Kane (1979) suggested the roles played by each hemisphere in a variety of different modes. For thinking, the right brain is described as deductive, divergent, intuitive, holistic, relating to concepts, simultaneity and geometry, whilst the left brain is described as inductive, convergent, segmented, logical and algebraic. Wheatley (1977; Wheatley et al., 1978) linked problem-solving styles with left and right brain specialisations. He described the right brain as all-at-once and gestalt and the left as one-at-a-time and serial. Wheatley also concluded that a good problem-solver achieves a smooth integration of the two modes of thinking.

The interpretation (or speculation) as to what the brain is doing is of some interest, in that it gives more credit to intuitive thinking. It seems somewhat dismissive to describe the 'global' thinker as intuitive, which seems to infer little conscious thought, when the intuitive process is probably based on rapid consideration of possibilities, experiences and knowledge, rather than being a sort of inspired, unconsidered guess.

# Cognitive Style in the Classroom

### Grasshoppers and inchworms

The work of Bath and Knox (1984) and Bath et al. (1986) on cognitive style arose from work and observations in the classroom, more specifically from teaching dyslexic children of secondary school age. It therefore has its roots in the observation of children with specific learning difficulties as they studied mathematics. Bath et al. labelled the two extremes of the continuum of cognitive styles as grassshoppers and inchworms. The characteristics of the two styles are summarised in Table 2.1 (Chinn, 1992) by looking at the three stages of solving a problem: identification, solving and verification.

### The teacher's role

Bath et al. (1986) investigated cognitive style by classifying answers to a series of selected mathematics questions, thus taking directly into account how a child actually does mathematics. One of the main recommendations of this book is the necessity for teacher and child to be flexible in their approach to mathematics – Krutetskii (1976) uses the wonderful word 'harmonious' to describe the blending of styles – yet to be aware that pupils (and teachers) may not always achieve this goal. Sharma (1989) commented on the need for teachers to be aware of cognitive style:

> All of us show and use different and unique mixtures of the two (personalities) but one approach is more dominant than the other in different individuals. And that is what the teacher should be aware of almost constantly.

Since you, the teacher, are usually in the controlling role, then the source and sanction for this flexibility must come predominantly from you. This situation is well expressed by Cobb (1991):

> We do not mean to imply that the teacher's beliefs are simply transferred to the student. Rather, the teacher has the authority to legitimize what is acceptable and to sanction what is not acceptable.

**Table 2.1**  Cognitive styles of the inchworm and the grasshopper

|  | *Inchworm* | *Grasshopper* |
|---|---|---|
| I. Analysing and identifying the problem | 1. Focuses on parts, attends to detail and separates | 1. Holistic, forms concepts and puts together |
|  | 2. Objective of looking at facts to determine useful formula | 2. Objective of looking at facts to determine an estimate of answer or range of restrictions |
| II. Methods of solving the problem | 3. Formula, recipe oriented | 3. Controlled exploration |
|  | 4. Constrained focusing using a single method or serially ordered steps along one route (Rifle approach), generally in one direction – forward | 4. Flexible focusing using multi-methods or paths, frequently occurring simultaneously (Shot gun approach), generally reversing or working back from an answer and trying new routes |
|  | 5. Uses numbers exactly as given | 5. Adjusts, breaks down/ builds up numbers to make an easier calculation |
|  | 6. Tending to add and multiply; resists subtraction and division | 6. Tending to subtract |
|  | 7. Tending to use paper and pencil to compute | 7. Tending to perform all computation mentally |
| III. Verification | 8. Verification unlikely; if done, uses same procedure or method | 8. Likely to verify; probably uses alternate procedure or method |

Source: Bath et al. (1986)

## The structure of mathematical abilities

Krutetskii (1976), in presenting a broad outline of the structure of mathematical abilities during school age, specifies a need for flexible thinking (and some skills which dyslexics may find hard). He specifies:

- The ability for logical thought in the sphere of quantitative and spatial relationships, number and letter symbols; the ability to think in mathematical symbols.

- The ability for rapid and broad generalization of mathematical objects, relations and operations.

- Flexibility of mental processes in mathematical activity.

- Striving for clarity, simplicity, economy and rationality of solutions.

- The ability for rapid and free reconstruction of the direction of a mental process, switching from a direct to a reverse train of thought.

- Mathematical memory (generalised memory for mathematical relationships), and for methods of problem solving and principles of approach.

These components are closely interrelated, influencing one another and forming in their aggregate a single integral syndrome of mathematical giftedness.

Although Krutetskii makes these observations concerning giftedness in mathematics, they are equally appropriate for competence. The reader can see where dyslexics may typically be at a disadvantage and where learning difficulties may create problems.

There are other sources of support for different learning styles (for example, and in more general terms, de Bono (1970)), but the emphasis of the remainder of this chapter is to paint a clearer picture of the background reasons for and consequences of different cognitive styles in mathematics.

**Learning styles**

To expand and clarify the picture of the two extremes of the cognitive style continuum, consider some mathematics problems and the solutions which an inchworm and a grasshopper might use. There is no implied value judgement on the two (extremes) of style. Indeed Kubrick and Rudnick (1980) suggested that teachers should encourage a wide variety of approaches, ideas and solutions. As has been already quoted, Krutetskii looks for a 'harmonious' approach.

# Examples

Some of the questions below are taken from the *Test of Cognitive Style in Mathematics* (Bath et al., 1986).

$2 \times 4 \times 3 \times 5$ (to be done mentally; no writing)

An inchworm will see first the 2 and the times sign. He tends not to overview the problem. Also he tends to take the problem 'literally', that is , if it says $2 \times 4 \times 3 \times 5$, then that is the order and it is not to be changed, and since 2 is an easy times table, he will begin: $2 \times 4 = 8$.

The next stage may be a little more challenging for times-table facts, but $8 \times 3 = 24$.

The last stage $(24 \times 5)$ may be too much of a challenge because of the load on short-term memory in multiplying 4 by 5, remembering that the unit digit is 0, carrying the 2, holding it in memory while multiplying 2 by

5, remembering the 2, knowing where to incorporate it, remembering the unit digit 0 and putting it all together to give 120. Some children will just say 'That's as far as I can get'.

A grasshopper, especially if he knows he has limited times-table knowledge, will overview the problem, reading through to the end to see if there are any short cuts or easy strategies or rearrangements. He may also be trying to get an estimate of the value of the answer.

He is likely to rearrange the problem to $(3 \times 4) \times (2 \times 5)$, i.e. $12 \times 10 = 120$. Thus he has taken a more global and flexible view of the question. In doing so he has reduced the demand on his times-table knowledge and the load on his short-term memory.

### Find three consecutive numbers which add up to make 60

An inchworm with some algebra skills will develop an equation;

Let the first number be $n$;

then the second number is $n + 1$

and the third number is $n + 2$.

So $n + (n + 1) + (n + 2) = 60$ which is then solved:

$3n + 3 = 60$

$3n = 60 - 3 = 57$

$n = 57/3$

$n = 19, \ n + 1 = 20, \ n + 2 = 21$.

The three numbers are 19, 20 and 21. The process is logical and sequential and is (effectively) independent of the value of the numbers involved; it will work for any similar problem. It takes the solution almost directly from the way the question is presented.

An inchworm without algebra skills will find it difficult to make a reasonable guess at a starting number. His subsequent adjustments to his guess will most probably be step by step, one at a time. So if his first guess is 10, his next guess is likely to be 11.

A grasshopper will start with a controlled exploration, leading to an estimate. He will see that the three numbers are approximately equal and that a good estimate of their value is given by $60/3 = 20$. It is only a short and easy step to 19, 20, 21. Again the strategy is holistic/global and peculiar to these numbers. It is an answer-oriented strategy.

**How many squares in Figure 2.2 are black?**

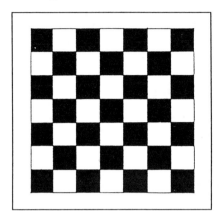

**Figure 2.2**

The pattern of $7 \times 7$ squares in Figure 2.2 is not equally divisible into black and white squares, which makes the problem less straightforward.

The inchworm will probably resort to counting each square. (He may initially count four across the top and four down the side and work on $4 \times 4$. Extreme inchworms would not see the obvious inaccuracy of this solution.) The inchworm is focusing on the parts of the square.

The grasshopper is holistic in his initial overview. The $7 \times 7$ squares make 49 and 'half' will be seen to be 25 since observation (of the corners or number of blacker rows) shows that the larger number of squares are black.

This problem illustrates the 'whole to parts' against the 'part to whole' contrast in the two styles.

**$37 + 85 + 36 + 19 + 43$**

The inchworm will rewrite the sum in vertical form:

3 7
8 5     The addition may be carried out with tallies to mark
3 6     progress and help the child keep count as he moves
1 9     down the numbers. The child is unlikely to use a pre-
4 3+    estimate or a check.

The inchworm will work in the order in which the numbers are given.

The grasshopper is likely to look for pairs and clusters of numbers which add to 10 or 20, e.g. in the unit column there is $7 + 3 = 10$ and $9 + 6 + 5 = 20$. In the tens column there is $3 + 3 + 4 = 10$ and from $8 + 1 + 3$ (carried from units) he can extract $8 + 2$, leaving 2. Answer 220.

The grasshopper will probably have already grouped 85 and 19 as a little over 100 and 36, 37 and 43 as a bigger bit over 100 – estimate 200 and a bit. He is using numbers as parts of a whole, where the whole is 10 or 100 or 1000. He is taking the numbers out of the order in which they are presented.

### Deductions from the examples

These examples are used to show how pupils with the two styles approach problems. Our experience of teaching dyslexic students leads us to some observations:

- there are pupils at the extremes of the continuum;
- an individual pupil may use both styles;
- the style an individual pupil uses can depend on the type of question or even on the level of difficulty of the same type of question;
- there are more inchworms than grasshoppers;
- inchworms with poor memory for basic facts are at risk in mathematics;
- grasshoppers need to learn how to document their work.

You have to be aware of these different styles and the fact that the child may not use the style he has been taught (Hart, 1978) or may, as Duffin (1991) observed, use his own method first and then diligently reproduce for the teacher the standard method he has been taught.

We could speculate which of the subskill deficits listed in Chapter 1 affect the way a child would solve such problems. For example, poor long-term memory for times-table facts could contribute to a grasshopper style, in that a child may have to overview and combine data in order to avoid facts that he cannot recall. What is clear is that the way a child (or adult) solves a question depends on the blend of deficits and strengths he brings to the problem. You can usually go a long way to finding out how a child solves a problem by asking the simple question, 'How did you do that?'. This interest (based on awareness), rather than a judgement, will be a major source of help for many pupils.

## Summary

Chinn and Bath (1993) are currently extending their work on cognitive style to include a measure of the learner's preference for abstract or concrete teaching methods and materials. This preference is presented as an extra dimension to cognitive style, so that the diagnostician (be he or she teacher, tutor, psychologist or parent) can be aware of how the child is more likely to learn mathematics. Sharma (1989) has already noted the different learning materials that quantitative and qualitative personalities prefer, distinguishing between discrete or quantitative materials (e.g. number lines) and continuous or qualitative materials (e.g. base-ten blocks).

If you are to teach effectively and diagnostically then you must be aware of and respond to the nature, variety and consequences of the child's strengths, weaknesses and cognitive style. An awareness that there is a range of cognitive styles in any teaching group can help you present a lesson more effectively and to a broader spectrum of learners.

# Chapter 3
# Testing and
# Diagnosis

If you are working with an individual student, you should use a diagnostic approach to teaching. You need to appraise the student's skills and deficits in mathematics. After some background considerations, this chapter suggests a testing procedure.

Chinn (1992, p. 23) has discussed the use of testing, in particular the benefits and disadvantages of norm-referenced and criterion-referenced tests. However, before returning to this discussion, we should step back and ask the obvious and fundamental question, 'Why test?'. Some of the answers to this question include:

- Parents may wish to know how their child's achievements compare with those of his peers.

- A teacher may wish to monitor the progress of his or her group and/or identify those who need extra help and/or collect data with which to stream groups.

- There may be a need to measure rates of progress.

- There may be some mandatory requirement to test.

- The test may be used to assess the ability of the child to progress to higher levels of study or to a new school.

- The test may be used to award a certificate recording a level of achievement (for example, GCSE or National Curriculum Key Stage 4).

- To provide information for an educational statement of special needs (which may be the same as the previous item).

- It may be used for diagnostic reasons (for example, to find the child's strengths, weaknesses, knowledge base and learning style).

It is understandable for a parent, or indeed a concerned educator, to wish to have an idea of the depth of a child's problems, measured in terms of a direct comparison with his peers. Tests which are 'normed' against a large population of children are used for these comparisons, for example the Vernon Miller Test, the NFER 8–12 Tests, the Profile of Mathematical Skills, the Basic Number Screening Test or the Wide Range Achievement Test (see the References and Appendix I for details). It is not the function of these tests to provide a diagnosis of 'dyslexic' problems. If the examiner wishes to derive a diagnostic profile of the child's strengths, weaknesses and learning style, additional testing will have to be done. The standardised test sets the baseline for the diagnosis.

Criterion-referenced tests are more diagnostic (by design) than norm-based tests. Interpretation of a criterion-based test can identify particular tasks that the child can and cannot do, but not necessarily his error patterns (Ashlock, 1982) or why he can or cannot do a particular task. Such tests can be lengthy if they are designed to be thorough and/or cover much ground (see Wilson and Sadowski, 1976). Ashcroft (see Appendix I) has designed a test based on items which tend to generate the errors typically made by dyslexics.

If these tests are used with groups, say as a class test, then the accurate interpretation of an individual child's errors can be uncertain and relies heavily on how much of his method the child has documented. Of course, if the test is administered to an individual, then diagnostic questioning can be used to supplement the written evidence. As in the *Test of Cognitive Style in Mathematics* (Bath et al., 1986), the key question is 'How did you do that?'. Careful, knowledgeable, well-timed and informed questioning is usually non-threatening.

## A Diagnostic Test Protocol

This diagnostic procedure, structured for a dyslexic child, links back, as does all the work in this book, to a knowledge of the child and what he brings to the subject. The procedure is designed to be appropriate to the child and to the mathematics he is likely to encounter. It also relates to the teaching strategies described in this book, indicating which are likely to be more effective for the child. Although the test items suggested here have been carefully selected, they may be modified to suit the individual. The structure and rationale of the test should, however, be followed.

The diagnostic procedure will examine the child's knowledge of basic facts, his levels of understanding of fundamental concepts (such as place value), his use of strategies (if any) and his learning style, and it should provide the examiner with enough information to construct a teaching programme appropriate to the child's needs.

The basic structure of the test protocol suggested below is designed to measure the child's present level of achievement and to ascertain why and in what ways the child is having difficulty. Although the basic premise must be that each child is a unique individual, there are certain common areas that are likely to create difficulty for the dyslexic (see Chapter 1). The protocol is designed to investigate these areas and to provide the examiner with a profile of the child's mathematical abilities. The test is aimed at early mathematics and therefore concentrates on numeracy. It is primarily designed for an age range from around 9 to about 13, depending on the extent of the deficit.

The test need not be given in one session, but may be spread over whatever time the examiner considers manageable for the child. Some items will be easier than others. The examiner should unobtrusively encourage the child to try his best.

## Structure of the Diagnostic Protocol

The test structure includes the following components:

- a norm-based test (see Appendix I);
- counting/adding on tasks and number bonds;
- times-table facts;
- place-value tasks;
- mathematics language;
- the four operations;
- money;
- word problems;
- attitude/anxiety.

### A norm-based (standardised) test

There are several to chose from (see the References and Appendix I for suggestions). The individual requirements of each examiner will probably reduce the choice. It is worth having several tests at the ready as many dyslexic children have a long history of being tested and may well have already done your first choice recently.

### Counting and adding on tasks

A good starting point is to scatter about 60 matchsticks or counters on a table top and ask the child to count them. The test is looking at one-to-one correspondence, speed of counting, accuracy and whether or not the child groups the counters/matchsticks and in what size of group.

The examiner can also ask the child to count the number of dots on a card, a task where he cannot handle and move the items he is counting. The dots can be presented in a regularly spaced line and then at random.

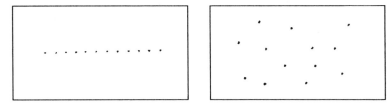

A series of fact cards may be made (on index cards) and used to check basic addition and subtraction skills. When testing for basic addition and subtraction fact knowledge and strategies, the examiner should also be aware of the Einstellung effect (Luchins, 1942), which is the lack of flexible interchange between operations (add, subtract, multiply and divide) and which is observed when a child stays with the original operation even after the operation sign has changed (a behaviour different to misreading signs).

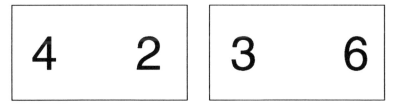

- 4 + 2 checks a basic, low number addition fact and whether the child counts on or just knows the answer.

- 3 + 6 checks as above and to see if the child changes the order to the easier counting on task of 6 + 3.

- 4 + 3 = [ ] introduces the child to the 'box' for an answer, a number to make the question 'right'. The examiner says, 'What number goes in the box to make the right answer?'.

- 5 + [ ] = 9 checks if the child is flexible enough in his knowledge of addition (and subtraction) to understand what is required, that is, does he count on or subtract 5 from 9 to obtain 4. The examiner asks 'What number goes in the box to make this sum right?'.

- 6 + 4 = [ ]. The number bonds for 10 are an important set of data to learn, so the child's level of knowing these facts needs to be checked.

- 'Can you write three more pairs of numbers that add up to 10, like 6 and 4?' Does the child immediately give you $4 + 6$, or does he have a strategy such as $9 + 1$, $8 + 2$, $7 + 3$?

- Give the child two 5p, six 2p and ten 1p coins and ask him to show you some ways of making 10p. Here the test is examining how many ways he produces 10p and whether they are to a system, e.g. $5 + 5$ to $5 + 2 + 2 + 1$ to $5 + 2 + 1 + 1 + 1$, etc.

- $10 = 7 + [\ ]$. Can the child use his number bonds for 10 in a different (subtraction) format?

- $8 + 7 = [\ ]$. Many children, even if they say they 'just know' the answer, can be gently persuaded to tell you exactly how they worked it out. Some children will simply count on, using their fingers or objects in the room. The finger movements may be very slight, so the examiner will have to be observant. Some children extend their limited lexicon of facts by interrelating number facts. So $8 + 7$ becomes 1 less than $2 \times 8$, i.e. $16 - 1 = 15$.

- $9 + 8 = [\ ]$, $9 + 6 = [\ ]$, $9 + 4 = [\ ]$. In asking this sequence (one at a time) the examiner is trying to see if the child has a consistent strategy for adding onto 9. Has the child started to see patterns?

- $17 - 8 = [\ ]$. Checks a problem similar to those above, but presented as a subtraction.

- $60 - 6 = [\ ]$. Can the child extend his number bonds for 10 to other 'ten' situations?

**Times-table facts**

Pritchard et al. (1989) found that dyslexics often knew the two times, five times and ten times tables, so the protocol can acknowledge this. The examiner can resort to straightforward questions, especially if he has established a good rapport with the child. He can simply ask 'Which of your times tables do you know?' and maybe prompt, 'The twos?'.

If the child says he does know the two times table the examiner should ask, 'What are seven twos, what is seven times two?'. The examiner must observe whether the child has instant recall or if he counts up 2, 4, 6, 8, 10, 12, 14 or if he uses a strategy, such as $5 \times 2$ and $2 \times 2$, added to make $7 \times 2$. Similar, careful diagnostic questioning can be used to establish a broad picture of the child's times-table knowledge.

The examiner may also wish to determine how many (if any) strategies the child uses to work out times-table facts. For example, if he knows that $2 \times 8 = 16$ does he add on a third 8 for $3 \times 8$, or if he knows $5 \times 8 = 40$, does he add another 8 to obtain $6 \times 8$? Another common strategy is to halve ten-times table facts to obtain five-times table facts. (A child who has developed his own strategies is more likely to be aware of the interrelationships between numbers.)

The commutative property is expressed as $a \times b = b \times a$, or in numbers, $7 \times 8 = 8 \times 7$, that is, it does not matter whether a rectangle is $9 \times 4$ or $4 \times 9$, the area is the same (36). The commutative property is useful knowledge and worth including in a test procedure. So a child may be asked to give the answer to $4 \times 8$ if he is told $8 \times 4 = 32$.

## Place value

The child is asked a series of questions. The numbers should be written on cards and shown to the child.

 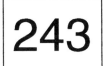

- If this number is fifty-six (56), what is this number? 243.

- What is this number? 8572.

- What is this number? 4016.

- Write the number (as digits) four thousand, two hundred and thirty three.

- Write the number sixteen thousand and seventeen.

- What is the value of each digit in this number? 5656

- Work out $14 \times 2$, $14 \times 20$, $14 \times 200$.

## The language of mathematics

- The child is asked to match the sign to the name. He can be told that there may be more than one name per sign. (The examiner needs two sets of cards, one set with four each of × + + − = /, the other set with add, divide, subtract, times, multiply, share, minus, plus, equals, same as, take away, more, less.)

- Make up an addition sum. The examiner may need to talk the child into this (e.g. $5 + 6 = 11$).

**Concepts/understanding**

- 'Explain what you understand by the word divide (or multiply).' The examiner will have different levels of expectation for this and may find that discussion can lead to a clearer picture of the child's under-standing of these deceptively simple concepts.

- 'Give me an estimate, an easier number to use, for 87.' The child may be bold enough to go to 100, but many will only go as far as 90. The examiner is looking to see if the child has understood the need to take an estimate to a number which is easy to use in calculations.

- Make up a word problem using in a mathematical way the word 'share'.

**The four operations $(+ - \times \div)$**

Ashlock's (1982) book *Error Patterns in Computation* introduces the idea of analysing a child's errors and then providing appropriate remedial instruction. Careful selection of computation items should give useful diagnostic information. This stage of the protocol also allows the exam-iner to introduce some criterion-referenced items.

*Addition*

These questions can be presented on a worksheet. The questions must be well spaced out and preferably ruled off from each other. The child can be asked to make an estimate for each question first. The use of a worksheet format does not preclude the continued use of the question, 'How did you do that?'.

- $\begin{array}{r} 36 \\ +21 \\ \hline \end{array}$  checks two digit plus two digit with no 'carrying'.

- $\begin{array}{r} 20 \\ +47 \\ \hline \end{array}$  checks adding to a zero.

- $\begin{array}{r} 357 \\ +469 \\ \hline \end{array}$  checks three digit plus three digit with two 'carries'.

- $8 + 5 + 7 + 5 + 1 + 9 + 2$ checks if the child uses number bonds for ten, rewrites the problem vertically, finger counts, tries to use memory, uses tallies, either to count each unit or as 'carries for tens'.

*Subtraction*

A further question sheet can be prepared, as in addition the examiner is looking at methods and errors instead of just whether the answers are right or wrong. Indeed both sets of questions were chosen to investigate the typical errors a dyslexic may make.

- 46      checks two digit minus two digit with no renaming. Renam-
  23 –    ing refers to changing 46 to 30 and 16, written $\overset{3\,1}{\cancel{4}\,6}$ .

- 73      checks two digit minus two digit with renaming.
  44 –

- 840     checks three digit minus three digit with subtraction from
  427 –   zero.

- 1000    checks use of renaming algorithm as opposed to rounding
  699 –   up the 699 to 700.

The questions are designed to investigate the typical errors dyslexics may make.

*Multiplication*

- 23      checks two digit times one digit with no carrying (with easy
  × 2     number facts).

- 37      checks two digit times one digit with carrying.
  × 2

- 23      relates to the first example to see if child can extend times
  × 20    two to times twenty.

- 42      checks two digit times two digit.
  × 22

- 514     checks three digit times three digit; also if the middle line is
  × 203   written as 000, i.e. 'blind' use of an algorithm.

Note that, although these examples are 'easy' they allow the child to demonstrate his ability to solve the problem without failing because he does not know times-table facts beyond two, five and ten. They also provide the examiner with information about the way the child solves basic multiplication problems and his error patterns.

*Division*

- $2\overline{)46}$    Checks two digit divided by one digit with no carrying.

- $2\overline{)74}$    Checks two digit divided by one digit with one carry.

- $5\overline{)56}$    Checks two digit divided by one digit with remainder (or decimal).

- $2\overline{)4008}$  Checks dividing into zeros.

Again the information required centres on methods and number concepts rather than basic fact knowledge.

## Word problems

Word problems should not be solely a test of reading ability, though the examiner needs to know if this is another barrier to success in mathematics. Again a clear worksheet should be written.

   The child is asked to read and solve the problems.

1. What is 7 add 3?

2. What is 49 minus 7?

3. Take 12 from 25.

4. If six boxes contain two pens each, how many pens altogether?

5. Mike has ten red pens, three paper clips and seven pencils. How many things can Mike use for writing?

6. Pat goes to the shop and buys two sweets at 5p each and ten sweets at 3p each. How much does he pay?

7. Sally and Kath have 22 model cars to share equally between them. How many do they each get?

- Questions 1 and 2 are the simplest and most straightforward.

- Question 3 reverses the order in which the numbers are to be subtracted.

- Question 4 mixes numbers as digits and numbers as words.

- Question 5 contains extraneous information.

- Question 6 has more than one stage.

- Question 7 is asking the child to divide and does not include any digits.

Thus each question probes a different aspect of the child's knowledge and abilities. His answers should give the examiner a good picture of the child's expertise with basic word problems. Although the questions are presented as a written exercise, once again the examiner can ask 'How did you do that?'.

## Money

Knowledge of money is a survival skill. It is also interesting to see how a child's ability to solve money problems compares with his ability to solve equivalent number problems. Later, the child's knowledge of money problems can be used, for example, to work with decimal fractions (see Chapter 10).

1. How many pence in one pound?

2. How much is half of a pound?

3. Show the child a card with £1.00 – 24p and ask him, 'How much change is there from a pound if a bar of chocolate costs 24p?'.

4. Show the child a card with £100 and £19 written on it and ask, 'If you have £100, how many computer games can you buy if each game costs £19? Do you have any change?'.

5. You have £5 and you want to buy four things which cost (show the child a card with £1.50 £2.50 75p 75p ). Have you enough money to buy all four things?

• Question 1 checks basic knowledge (essential to complete the other questions).

• Question 2 is asking if the child has absorbed what 50p is.

• Question 3 is 'real' life mathematics and looks at division.

• Question 4 is asking if the child has a concept of the value of money. Does he know that £100 is an identifiable amount of money.

• Question 5 is looking at another typical 'shopping' exercise.

# Attitude and anxiety

It may also help and encourage the child if he is asked questions such as the following:

• 'How do you like mathematics?'

• 'Do you think you are any good at mathematics?'

• 'Which bits of maths do you like best?'

• 'Are there any areas where you think you could do with a little help?'

## Summary of the Test Protocol

The answers to the questions combined with a knowledge of the way the child solves each question should provide the examiner with a comprehensive picture of what the child can do and how he does it, i.e. the examiner has a measure of the child's basic knowledge and his use of numeracy skills. The child's cognitive style can be deduced from such behaviours as whether he finger counts to solve $8 + 7$ or if he uses $(2 \times 8) - 1$, his estimate for 87, or how he solves $1000 - 699$. Alternatively a cognitive style test can be used. As well as providing a picture of the child's strengths and weaknesses, the protocol helps you as the teacher to obtain a clearer idea as to what strategies the child is likely to find easy and which he will find harder to absorb.

# Chapter 4
# Concept of
# Number

## Introduction

When a child has problems learning the basic facts of number, then his problems may be compounded by his consequent failure to develop an understanding of the values and interrelationships of numbers (of course, it does not automatically follow that a child who successfully rote learns the basic facts will develop an understanding of numbers). It is important that any child should develop a 'feel' or 'facility' for number, i.e. he needs to learn

- a sense of the size or value of a number;

- recognition of the other numbers which it is near to;

- how near it is to other numbers, particularly 'key' numbers such as tens, hundreds, etc.;

- whether it is larger or smaller, and by roughly how much;

- its relationship to other numbers (twice as big, etc.).

For children with learning difficulties in mathematics, the development of this facility is a likely alternative route to coping with early numeracy. Their early failure to learn basic number facts can keep them from the extent and quality of experiences needed to develop number concept.

This chapter looks at the very early stages of number work. These are stages where a dyslexic child may have started to fail. Thus, even an older child may need work to recover the experiences he has not taken on board earlier. As with much of the material in this book, the work described may not be age-specific. As tutor/teacher, you need to adjust the style and approaches of your presentation of the work to avoid patronising the child.

## Early Recognition of Numbers and Their Values

A *small* number of objects can usually be recognised instantaneously by using a visual sense of number, so that a child seeing two different clusters of, say, four spots will recognise them as the same quantity. This ability disappears with larger numbers (though some children have been able to extend the skill to remarkably large numbers).

Slightly larger numbers may be more quickly recognised if:

1. The objects are arranged in a recognisable pattern, or

2. The number can be seen as a combination of other numbers. Thus, even at this early stage of development, the child can be introduced to the use of patterns and interrelationships.

So, for example, nine can be shown as

or                    (domino pattern).

Teachers (or parents) can also introduce certain special numbers that can be used as landmarks, reference points or stepping stones towards understanding other numbers. For example, nine can be seen as one less than ten, and twelve can be seen as two more than ten. Thus ten is introduced as a useful number.

## The Language of Mathematics

In this chapter, we use the word 'number' to mean one of the following:

- the mathematical symbol for the number, e.g. 8;

- the written form of the number word, e.g. eight;

- the sound of a number word, e.g. ate (phonetic: āt).

So already we have three interpretations of even such a basic word as 'number'.

For most of the dyslexics we teach, the problem of mathematics as a 'foreign' language becomes particularly acute when there is a necessity to write numbers down. The situation is exacerbated by the conventions of place value (base ten).

# Early Number Work

### Sorting/classifying

An important mathematical pre-skill is the ability to differentiate objects and group together those with common attributes, such as colour, size or function. This activity is the first stage towards counting the objects in a set.

The number zero is an important concept to introduce, even at this early stage. It can be introduced here to represent the complete absence of any objects in the set (or group). This early exposure is important and quite easy to introduce in a clear way to a child.

### Correspondence between sets of objects

Understanding that two sets contain the same number of objects can be achieved by matching each object from the first set with each object from the second. If there are any objects left after such a matching process, then one set contains more objects and the other contains fewer objects.

This level of understanding allows sets of objects to be compared, even though the actual number in neither set is established. This acts as an early introduction to the concept of 'more than' and 'less than'. The same approach can be extended to compare more than two sets and thus the idea of rank orders.

The idea of comparing two sets can be extended to record the number of objects in the first set by using 'tallies' in the second set. The tallies should be a familiar, standard set of objects such as fingers or marks recorded on paper, one tally for each object,

e.g. 1, 11, 111, 1111, 11111, 111111, 1111111, 11111111

1, 11, 111, 1111, 1̶1̶1̶1̶1̶, 1̶1̶1̶1̶1̶1̶, 1̶1̶1̶1̶1̶11, 1̶1̶1̶1̶1̶111

### Correspondence between objects and numbers: counting

*Stage 1*

Introducing the number words and number symbols gives, in effect, abstract sets, which can be matched with sets of actual objects. For example, when the set of three objects is seen to correspond with the symbol '3', we begin to call the number of objects three.

It can then be seen that if the objects are counted in any different order, the correspondence shows that there are still three. Furthermore, if other sets of different objects are also seen to correspond with 3, then the relationship of a constant 'three-ness' for the two 'different' sets can be developed. Another important move forward comes if the child can be encouraged to explore the arrangement of objects within a set to discover that the number is conserved even though the arrangement is different. In this way the child learns the interrelationship of numbers, e.g. $3 = 2 + 1$ or $1 + 2$.

## Stage 2

At this stage the child is starting to link together the objects, the symbol for the number of objects, and the word (sight and sound) for the number, and the 'break down' of the number (Table 4.1).

**Table 4.1**

| Objects | 1 | 11 | 111 | 1111 | 11111 | 111111 | 1111111 | 11111111 | 111111111 |
|---|---|---|---|---|---|---|---|---|---|
| Number symbols | 1 | 2 | 3 | 4 | 5 | 6 | 7 | 8 | 9 |
| Words/sounds | One | Two | Three | Four | Five | Six | Seven | Eight | Nine |

It is necessary for the number symbols and sounds in the above table to be known by heart. The exact spelling of the number words is of less importance (and less achievable) for children with this type of learning difficulty. The ARROW strategy (Lane, 1992) may well be of use to help achieve this target. ARROW is a multisensory learning and teaching approach developed in schools and researched under the auspices of Somerset County Council and the University of Exeter. ARROW uses a child's own voice, the self-voice, to develop rapidly skills central to reading, spelling, speaking and listening. ARROW is an acronym for Aural–Read–Respond–Oral–Written in which the self-voice, replayed on tape, is linked to writing, listening and speech skills in a series of processes involving spelling, comprehension and reading books.

## Stage 3

Counting can be used to associate the movement from object to object with a movement to the next number. In the early stages, while counting aloud, a child cannot always synchronise these movements and it may help if he counts against a regular rhythm or beat (e.g. a metronome).

## Stage 4

The extension of the skill of counting forwards to the skill of counting backwards is not easy for the dyslexic child. More practice in the reverse operation of removing one object at a time while counting the numbers backwards will almost certainly be needed.

*Stage 5*

*The Number Line* (Figure 4.1) is useful at all levels of mathematics. Here it associates each extra mark with the next number and confers an evenness and proportionality on the counting process. It also establishes the order of the numbers, as well as the convention of increasing to the right and decreasing to the left. Furthermore, the regular spacing of the numbers begins the connection between numbers and length. This is reinforced by using apparatus of the Dienes and Cuisenaire types.

```
0
  |__|__|__|__|__|__|__|__|__|_____
     1  2  3  4  5  6  7  8  9
```

**Figure 4.1**   The Number Line

*Stage 6*

Some link between the symbols and the values of low numbers can be (somewhat artificially) drawn by stylisation of the number symbols. This may be a useful mnemonic for some children, e.g.

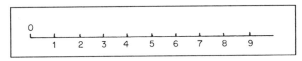

For this stylisation the number of bold strokes suggests the number of objects.

## Visual Sense of Number

Experiments can show that the visual sense of numbers is limited to about five or six. That is to say, most children will immediately recognise the number of objects in sets of one, two, three, four, five or six (without time for counting). This seems to imply that children have an in-built 'feel' for the sizes or values of these numbers.

From about six objects onwards, the visual sense of number is exhausted and the objects have to be counted, unless there are other clues in the arrangement of the objects. In other words, the child has to use a one-to-one correspondence, treating each number as a separate identity; he begins to relate numbers, build them up and see constituent parts.

## Visual Clues to Number Concept

Numbers can more easily be 'assessed' if they form a recognisable pattern or if they can be seen as a combination of simpler numbers (this can be done in the early stages without a formal understanding of addition or multiplication). At this stage such an exercise adds further reinforcement to the idea of breaking down and building up numbers. The work can then be extended to bigger numbers, as shown in Figure 4.2. Many of the numbers are instantly recognisable through their patterns, familiar from dice and dominoes.

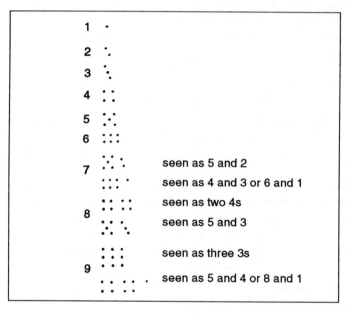

**Figure 4.2** Breaking down and building up numbers

Any attempt to 'standardise' on a particular version is likely to be counterproductive, because each child will feel happiest with the version that suits him individually. Our experience is that children have started to build up their own idiosyncratic lexicons of facts and links. The best version is the one that works for a particular child, although sometimes a little intrusion helps to rationalise and organise the child's ideas.

## Number Bonds

The number bonds (for sums below ten) are fundamental in aiding number concept. The preceding work has built up to this formal presentation of number facts. Knowledge of the number bonds is also important when addition is tackled formally. There are therefore two important reasons why they should be understood and learned at this early stage. The following are likely to be the most useful:

|        | A         | B         | C         | D         |
|--------|-----------|-----------|-----------|-----------|
| 2 as   | 1 and 1   |           |           |           |
| 3 as   | 2 and 1   |           |           |           |
| 4 as   | 3 and 1   | 2 and 2   |           |           |
| 5 as   | 4 and 1   | 3 and 2   |           |           |
| 6 as   | 5 and 1   | 4 and 2   | 3 and 3   |           |
| 7 as   | 6 and 1   | 5 and 2   | 4 and 3   |           |
| 8 as   | 7 and 1   | 6 and 2   | 5 and 3   | 4 and 4   |
| 9 as   | 8 and 1   | 7 and 2   | 6 and 3   | 4 and 5   |

Column A gives practice at adding 1, column B at adding 2, column C at adding 3 and column D at adding 4.

Practice can, for example, be scheduled in the following ways:

- adding 1 to each number from 1 to 8;

- adding every number from 2 to 7 to the number 2;

- adding the numbers randomly;

- adding numbers in every possible way to make a given sum, such as 7.

The practice can be supported by using 'concrete' materials:

1. Any form of counters that remain separate, so that the child sees the 'ones' in each part and the resultant whole.

2. Blocks, like centicubes, which can be joined together and separated, so that the child starts to see the numbers holistically.

3. Cuisenaire-type rods, each number represented by a different length and colour, so that the child visualises the 'sizes' of the numbers.

4. A number line, which links the numbers to a sense of proportionality.

5. The child can use two spinners which can take any value from 1 to 8, or an eight-sided dice (used in conjunction with 1–4 if necessary).

An important consequence of this work should be the establishment of the commutative law, which states that the order in which the numbers are added does not affect the answer, i.e. $5 + 2 = 2 + 5$ $(= 7)$.

You will need to establish the law by reminding and organising the child to see the logic of the demonstrations he has just undertaken.

This latter concept, plus that of number bonds and the results of the practice described above are all summarised as shown below:

| + | 1 | 2 | 3 | 4 | 5 | 6 | 7 | 8 |
|---|---|---|---|---|---|---|---|---|
| 1 | 2 | 3 | 4 | 5 | 6 | 7 | 8 | 9 |
| 2 | 3 | 4 | 5 | 6 | 7 | 8 | 9 |   |
| 3 | 4 | 5 | 6 | 7 | 8 | 9 |   |   |
| 4 | 5 | 6 | 7 | 8 | 9 |   |   |   |
| 5 | 6 | 7 | 8 | 9 |   |   |   |   |
| 6 | 7 | 8 | 9 |   |   |   |   |   |
| 7 | 8 | 9 |   |   |   |   |   |   |
| 8 | 9 |   |   |   |   |   |   |   |

This table can be used for reference by the child and as a compact source from which to memorise the data.

## Place Value

The use of base ten and the consequent place value of numbers are conventions. The most frequent (and predictable) difficulty that occurs is that the child does not understand that the value of a number depends on its place in a group of numbers. This difficulty is not to be confused with the transposition of numbers (e.g. 34 for 43). There are also some problems with misunderstanding the language of these conventions. Many subsequent problems can be traced back to a lack of understanding of place value. It therefore needs careful attention.

### Grouping in tens

The number ten owes its significance to the number of our fingers and their use in counting. Ten retains its significance as a collective unit in the written symbols we use for numbers, so we have ten fingers and ten different number symbols. When we ran out of fingers, we had to use something else (a second person's fingers for example), so when we ran out of number symbols we had to use a second, additional symbol (in another column or place).

The following approach attempts to show a logical connection between a number of objects and the symbols used to write the numbers. The approach moves from the concrete to the abstract, 'foreign language', written form in progressively more abstact/representative forms.

### Step 1. Physically grouping

Objects do not naturally form themselves into groups of ten. Practice in doing this can be the first step towards understanding. The type of exercise here is simply to provide a group of items and let the child group them in tens. What the child sees are groups of tens which are numerically proportional to their value (Figure 4.3).

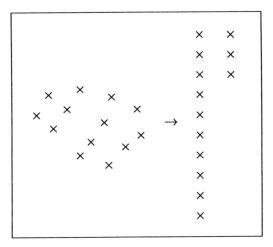

**Figure 4.3**  Physically grouping

### Step 2. Using counting blocks

Certain types of counting blocks (especially Dienes/base-ten blocks) have a different block for ten, which is in direct proportion to the length of ten unit blocks (Figure 4.4).

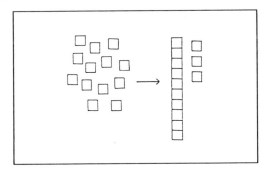

**Figure 4.4**  Counting blocks

### Step 3. Using money

Although a 10p coin is physically larger than a 1p coin, it is not proportionally ten times bigger. It is a different colour. The use of money therefore brings further progress towards abstraction (Figure 4.5 a).

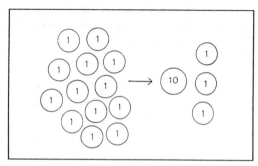

**Figure 4.5a**  Using money

## Step 4. Using written tally symbols

The use of different tally symbols for ten and 1, such as the ancient Egyptian Λ and I, gives a written symbol parallel for the money activity above (Figure 4.5b).

IIIIIIIIIIIII  →  ∩III          IIIIIIIII
                              IIIIIIIIIIII  →  ∩∩III

**Figure 4.5b**  Using tally symbols

Another suitable manipulative type of object here is bundles of ten cocktail sticks and single cocktail sticks. The material retains proportionality, but emphasises the 'collecting together' of units into tens.

## Step 5. Recording in words

Writing numbers down can be achieved using the words 'Tens' and 'Ones' as labels (Figure 4.6).

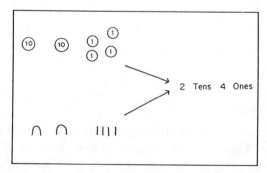

**Figure 4.6** Recording in words

## Step 6. Using headings instead of labels

Writing these labelsfor each number is inefficient and time consuming, but using them as headings (Figure 4.7) saves some of this effort while leaving a clear reminder of the existence and value of the number places. Later we will use place value cards to help maintain the concept during addition and subtraction.

|         |        |   | Tens | Ones |
|---------|--------|---|------|------|
| 2 Tens  | 4 Ones | → | 2    | 4    |
| 6 Tens  | 9 Ones | → | 6    | 9    |
| 5 Tens  | 2 Ones | → | 5    | 2    |
| 8 Tens  | 3 Ones | → | 8    | 3    |

**Figure 4.7**  Using headings

## Step 7. Omission of the headings

Eventually, the headings can be dropped when they are 'understood' to be there, defining the place value of the digit (Figure 4.8).

| 2 | 4 |
|---|---|
| 6 | 9 |
| 5 | 2 |
| 8 | 3 |

**Figure 4.8**  Omission of headings

## Tens alone

When we write 10, we mean 1 ten and 0 ones. In some number systems, it would be redundant to mention the 0 ones, because zero means there are no objects there. Place value uses fixed relative positions (reinforced by column headings where place value is less well understood). So an understanding of the role of 0 as marking that a particular 'place' is empty is essential, as is its role of maintaining the 'place' of the other digits. One good way of demonstating this with children is to make each child a place value and his fingers the digits, so that 30 looks like Figure 4.9. The teacher can discuss with the children why the second (unit) child is needed to demonstrate 30.

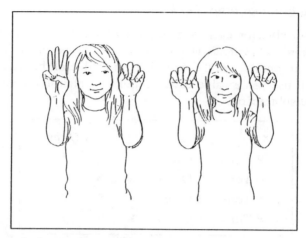

**Figure 4.9  Hands showing place value**

Figure 4.10 shows three ways of depicting four tens. They must be identified as tens, classified, counted and recorded together. The 0 in the written version 40 makes it quite clear that:

- the 4 objects are tens, and

- there are no ones.

In the spoken form, ten became abbreviated to -ty. Hence six tens became sixty, etc. Although it is obviously incorrect and contrived there is some good teaching value in the use of 'tenty' for one hundred. For example, it is a logical extension of the pattern of the other '-ty' numbers and helps the child realise something new is happening if we change the rule/pattern to a new word – hundred. It is also useful in subtraction if renaming from the hundred column is used.

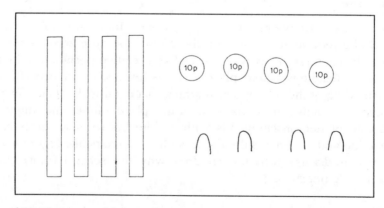

**Figure 4.10**  Three ways of depicting four tens

## Grouping in hundreds

After 10, 20, 30, 40, 50, 60, 70, 80, 90, it is impossible to record any more tens in the tens column (we have run out of number symbols again). If the example used 10p pieces, there would also be an argument against having too many coins. The solutions to the two situations are parallel: we use another collective unit, hundred (in another column), or we use another coin, £1. In each case, the hundred can be seen as 10 tens. Cocktail sticks may again be used here, especially if available in boxes of 100. In Figure 4.11 the number 237 is represented in various ways.

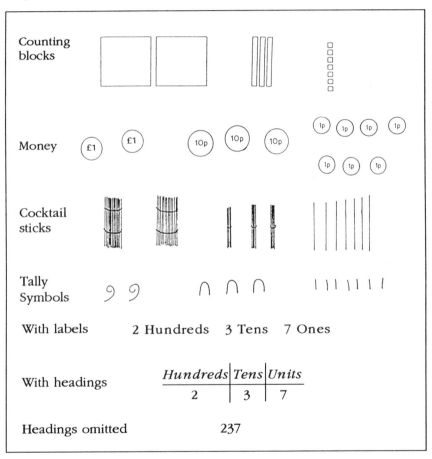

**Figure 4.11**  Representations of the number 237

## Grouping in thousands

Thousand is the next collective unit, constituted from 10 hundreds. The next collective units are ten thousand and hundred thousand. The analogues of the counting blocks, money, tally symbols and labels are less effective in contributing to an understanding of numbers above a thousand, though discussions about how many ten-base thousand blocks would be needed to construct these higher value numbers are helpful. Fortunately, if place value has been properly understood up to this point, further extension of the system offers no further fundamental problems.

Certain large numbers with thousands can cause problems because of language, the word hundred being repeated in hundred thousand and/or the large number of digits, many of which can be zeros. For example, the number two hundred and six thousand and fifty can be incorrectly written as 200600050, 2006050, 20600050, 2060050, etc. It can be helpful to consider the number in two parts: the thousands separate from the rest, which must fill three places (for hundreds, tens and ones) set aside in advance, e.g. for the above number the first step would be 206---, then 206-50, then 206050.

## Millions

The collective unit million virtually completes the picture. The first new word after thousand, it is probably best considered as a 1000 thousand. Again consideration of the space occupied by a thousand 'thousand' blocks can help the concept. This space is, of course, the space occupied by a metre cube.

Some children can cope with exercises such as finding how high a pile of a million pound coins would be. Ideas like this make useful investigations which can be used to develop concepts of large numbers.

## Reminders

At this stage any doubt about a number will usually be clarified by the reintroduction of column headings.

## Diagnostic ideas

Questions of the following kinds can be used for practice, and for diagnosing difficulties:

- What is the value of the 7 in the number 4725?

- Write in figures thirty thousand and five.

- Write in words 12065.

- Write down the largest and smallest three-digit numbers you can make with the three digits 2, 6 and 9.

## Number Bonds for 10

Because of its universal importance, it is essential for a child to have a good concept of 10. It is worth making a special study of the number bonds for 10 and, if at all possible, helping the child to learn these facts. This is said with the clear understanding that rote learning is extraordinarily difficult for most dyslexics, but then, if the child does have to learn facts, let those facts be the ones with the most value/mileage. There are several illustrations and exercises which can be used to help the child understand and visualise these facts.

$$9 + 1 \atop 8 + 2 \Big\}$$ Especially useful for estimation/mental arithmetic purposes

$7 + 3$

$6 + 4$

$5 + 5$ ←Some children readily understand and remember 'doubles';
$4 + 6$     5 is exactly half of 10

$3 + 7$

$2 + 8$

$1 + 9$

All the different ways of making 10 can be found, for example, by:

- joining together 10 centicubes, then breaking them up in various ways;
- laying down a Cuisenaire rod for 10, then laying down beside it combinations of other rods to give the same length;
- using an abacus;
- using coins.

Diagrams like those in Figures 4.12 and 4.13 can help the memory.

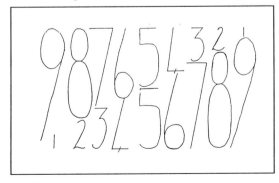

**Figure 4.12**

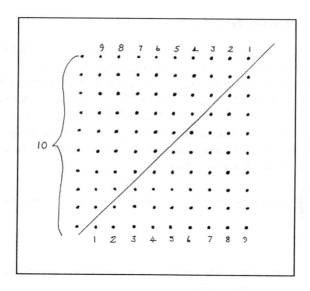

**Figure 4.13**

# Numbers near to 10, 100 or 1000

Ten, hundred and thousand are major 'landmarks' and reference points in the base-10 system.

- From them, steps outwards can give meaning to numbers nearby, above or below. For example, the number 8 is just less than 10, and the number 1100 is just over 1000.

- Later, a question like $4 \times 98$ can be seen as just below $4 \times 100$. This can give the approximate answer 'just below 400', or can form the starting point for estimation work and (mental) calculations of the form

$$4 \times 98 = 4 \times 100 - 4 \times 2$$

$$= 400 - 8$$

$$= 392.$$

- A number of diagrams are given in Figures 4.14, 4.15 and 4.16, which give a picture of the relative sizes/positions of the numbers 10, 100, 1000 and of the numbers near to them.

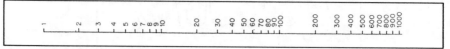

**Figure 4.14** Pseudo-logarithmic scale

*Advantages/Disadvantages*

The pseudo-logarithmic scale in Figure 4.14 shows all the numbers 10, 100, 1000, on the same line, but the unequal gaps between the numbers would confuse some children, and it is difficult to read in parts.

The number lines with periodic curves in Figure 4.15 show the relative positions clearly, but relating each line to the others may cause problems.

On the number blocks shown in Figure 4.16, the positions and the numbers are quite clear. However, the number 1000 cannot be included on the same diagram.

The diagram, or combination of diagrams, which a child follows most easily is again the best alternative. All this is of course preceded by work using as many concrete materials as appropriate (e.g. money, Dienes, metre rule). The diagrams are somewhat demanding conceptually, but they do summarise a concept and spatial presentation that is difficult to do otherwise.

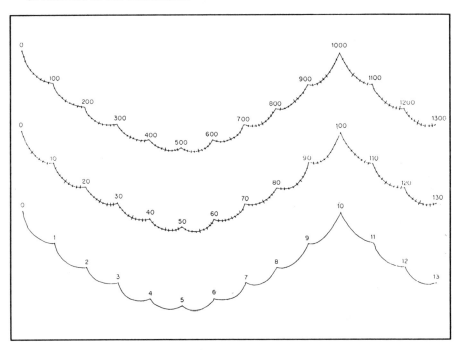

**Figure 4.15** Number lines with periodic curves

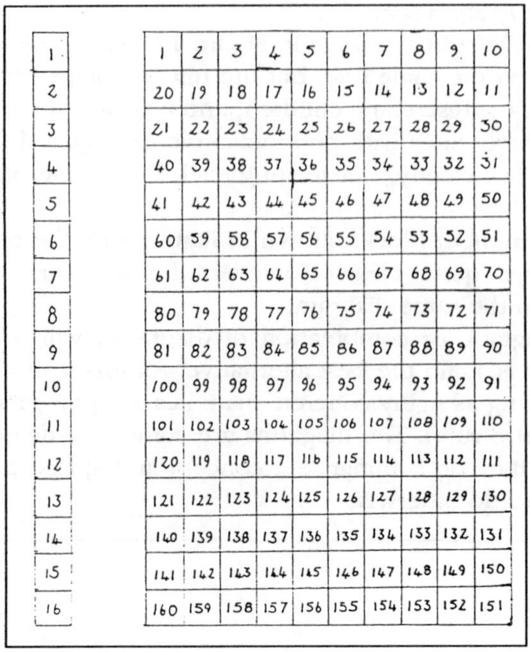

| | | | | | | | | | | |
|---|---|---|---|---|---|---|---|---|---|---|
| 1 | 1 | 2 | 3 | 4 | 5 | 6 | 7 | 8 | 9 | 10 |
| 2 | 20 | 19 | 18 | 17 | 16 | 15 | 14 | 13 | 12 | 11 |
| 3 | 21 | 22 | 23 | 24 | 25 | 26 | 27 | 28 | 29 | 30 |
| 4 | 40 | 39 | 38 | 37 | 36 | 35 | 34 | 33 | 32 | 31 |
| 5 | 41 | 42 | 43 | 44 | 45 | 46 | 47 | 48 | 49 | 50 |
| 6 | 60 | 59 | 58 | 57 | 56 | 55 | 54 | 53 | 52 | 51 |
| 7 | 61 | 62 | 63 | 64 | 65 | 66 | 67 | 68 | 69 | 70 |
| 8 | 80 | 79 | 78 | 77 | 76 | 75 | 74 | 73 | 72 | 71 |
| 9 | 81 | 82 | 83 | 84 | 85 | 86 | 87 | 88 | 89 | 90 |
| 10 | 100 | 99 | 98 | 97 | 96 | 95 | 94 | 93 | 92 | 91 |
| 11 | 101 | 102 | 103 | 104 | 105 | 106 | 107 | 108 | 109 | 110 |
| 12 | 120 | 119 | 118 | 117 | 116 | 115 | 114 | 113 | 112 | 111 |
| 13 | 121 | 122 | 123 | 124 | 125 | 126 | 127 | 128 | 129 | 130 |
| 14 | 140 | 139 | 138 | 137 | 136 | 135 | 134 | 133 | 132 | 131 |
| 15 | 141 | 142 | 143 | 144 | 145 | 146 | 147 | 148 | 149 | 150 |
| 16 | 160 | 159 | 158 | 157 | 156 | 155 | 154 | 153 | 152 | 151 |

**Figure 4.16** Number blocks

## Summary

This chapter has looked at the concept of numbers and their values, concentrating on place value. The remaining chapters will continue to develop number concept and facility by extending the child's experiences into the interrelationships of numbers. What is important at this stage is that the child has some clear ideas as to the values of the low numbers, an understanding of number bonds in the light of conservation of number and the commutative law, and a clear concept of place value. This knowledge will form a good base for the remaining development.

# Chapter 5
# Addition and Subtraction: Basic Facts

## Introduction

If you ask dyslexic children to add 8 and 7 and explain how they reached their answer you will get a selection of methods depending on each child's experiences and own idiosyncratic ideas, for example:

- Counting on: the child simply starts at 8 and counts on 7 (using his fingers or counting on objects in the room).

- Using 10: the child breaks 7 into $2 + 5$, uses the 2 with the 8 to make 10, then adds on 5, or works via $7 + 3$.

- Using doubles: the child uses $(2 \times 8) - 1$ or $(2 \times 7) + 1$.

- Straight recall: the child 'just knows'.

In this chapter we will look at strategies for working out basic facts efficiently and in a way that enhances number concept and facility with number. We are assuming that a child will have great difficulty in rote-learning the facts and, if he should succeed, holding those facts for more than a few hours. Each child therefore needs strategies to use when his memory fails him and leaves him with no way to obtain an answer. Some strategies are going to be used in their entirety, but others can be mastered to the stage where they become memory 'hooks' and are only used in part to supplement a half-known fact.

The strategy of counting on is not an effective strategy beyond counting on 1 or 2. It is a method that requires too much time to operate and it tends, therefore, to be susceptible to poor short-term memory. It is also susceptible to counting errors. Furthermore, it does not support number concept, nor the relationships between, and patterns of, numbers. Strategies which use number relationships are advocated wherever possible.

It is easy to underestimate just how much early experience and information a dyslexic student has missed, which makes it difficult to know

47

how far back to go when starting a teaching programme. One of the key ideas that this chapter advocates is the breaking down and building up of numbers. So, if a child did not receive and absorb work such as looking at 6 as in Figure 5.1, then strategies which suggest that $8 + 6$ can be added as $(8 + 2) + 4$ will be less easy to teach (or learn). As ever, you have to 'read' the child to know how much material to provide. (Ashlock et al. (1983) provide an excellent range of teaching ideas to develop and reinforce algorithms and concepts.)

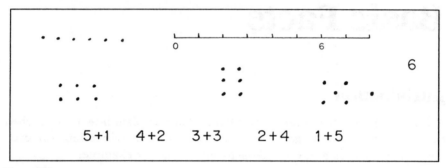

**Figure 5.1**

# Strategies for Learning/Remembering the Addition Facts

The basic addition facts from 0 to 10 can be arranged in a square (Figure 5.2; see also times-table facts). This gives the child a task of rote-learning 121 facts or developing strategies for as many of these facts as possible.

The procedure for addressing the addition facts task is similar in technique to that used for times tables. It uses patterns, the interrelationships between numbers and the ability to break down and build up numbers. It builds on strategies which the children themselves use, but organises and rationalises idiosyncratic ideas. The structure of a square of facts gives some motivation in that initial gains can be shown quickly and strategies are less individual, that is, they can be more flexible and extensible.

### The zero facts: +0

$n + 0$ and $0 + n$ can be established using, for example, counters in boxes.

- An empty box is shown to the child and, after discussion about the contents and zero, 0 is written on the board or a sheet of paper.

- Five counters are added to the box. $+ 5$ is written on the board/paper, giving $0 + 5$.

| + | 0 | 1 | 2 | 3 | 4 | 5 | 6 | 7 | 8 | 9 | 10 |
|---|---|---|---|---|---|---|---|---|---|---|---|
| 0 | 0 | 1 | 2 | 3 | 4 | 5 | 6 | 7 | 8 | 9 | 10 |
| 1 | 1 | 2 | 3 | 4 | 5 | 6 | 7 | 8 | 9 | 10 | 11 |
| 2 | 2 | 3 | 4 | 5 | 6 | 7 | 8 | 9 | 10 | 11 | 12 |
| 3 | 3 | 4 | 5 | 6 | 7 | 8 | 9 | 10 | 11 | 12 | 13 |
| 4 | 4 | 5 | 6 | 7 | 8 | 9 | 10 | 11 | 12 | 13 | 14 |
| 5 | 5 | 6 | 7 | 8 | 9 | 10 | 11 | 12 | 13 | 14 | 15 |
| 6 | 6 | 7 | 8 | 9 | 10 | 11 | 12 | 13 | 14 | 15 | 16 |
| 7 | 7 | 8 | 9 | 10 | 11 | 12 | 13 | 14 | 15 | 16 | 17 |
| 8 | 8 | 9 | 10 | 11 | 12 | 13 | 14 | 15 | 16 | 17 | 18 |
| 9 | 9 | 10 | 11 | 12 | 13 | 14 | 15 | 16 | 17 | 18 | 19 |
| 10 | 10 | 11 | 12 | 13 | 14 | 15 | 16 | 17 | 18 | 19 | 20 |

**Figure 5.2.** The square of facts

- The child counts the number of counters in the box, 5.
- The written form now has $0 + 5 = 5$.

A similar procedure may be used to deduce $5 + 0 = 5$. Careful and emphasised use of language is needed if later confusion with $\times 0$ facts is to be pre-empted.

This establishes 21 facts, though, as is ever the case, an unusual presentation of a 'known' fact may confuse the child. A typical error occurs in addition sums such as

$$
\begin{array}{r}
356 \\
+ 30 \\
\hline
380 \\
\end{array}
$$

### Adding on 1 (and 2)

This can be introduced by asking the child to look at a number line and handle counters, so that he sees, say, $4 + 1$ as one move on the number line, i.e. a move to the next number. He can also experience a move to the next number by counting the addition with counters or, say, unifix cubes. The child has to 'see' the process as simply moving to the next number.

A very similar argument applies to adding 2, though the child may have to physically count on the two numbers. This should still be quick

and accurate. A knowledge of the even and odd numbers will support
this operation. The child can practise counting in twos, starting from different numbers. The child will then need to spend some time looking at
facts such as $1 + 9$ and $2 + 7$, with the teacher talking him into the commutative property of $1 + n = n + 1$ and teaching that it is quicker, less
prone to error and more effective to count the smaller onto the bigger
number.

If this can be accomplished, then 36 more fact squares can be shaded
in, a total of 57, leaving 64 to go.

## Adding to 10; adding on 10

It is often the case when working with dyslexics that a lesson has more
than one goal. The subsidiary goal is usually a review of a previously
'learned' (and perhaps 'forgotten') fact or concept. In this case the forgotten concept is likely to be that 10 represents 1 in the tens place-value column and zero in the units place-value column (i.e. it is an empty
column). If this is re-established, then adding on to 10 is taking the child
back to the first family of basic addition facts, i.e. $n + 0$ and $0 + n$ and
extending it to $n + 10$ and $10 + n$.

A teaching idea is to use a place-value card and discuss and do the
addition in symbols and with counters. There is some benefit in using 1p
and 10p coins or base-ten 'longs' and 'units' because they clearly illustrate
the difference between unit and ten values.

The visual pattern is

$$10 + 1 = 11$$
$$10 + 2 = 12$$
$$10 + 3 = 13$$
$$10 + 4 = 14, \text{ etc.}$$

The tens digit (1) does not change, but the units digit becomes the same
as the added number, $10 + d = 1d$ (not algebra!). An extra difficulty
sometimes arises from the unfortunate fact that the names of the numbers
from 11 to 19, unlike subsequent decades, have the unit digit named first,
e.g. seventeen. This also makes the aural pattern less consistent.

If this series of facts is understood then the task has reduced to 49
facts.

## Use of doubles

For addition facts, children often know the doubles (similarly, in multiplication they often know the squares) and also use them to derive other
addition facts, for example, $8 + 7$ is often seen as double 8 less 1 (and
sometimes as double 7 plus 1).

Two columns of counters provide a good representation of the derivation of these facts. Cuisenaire rods are also useful, e.g. two seven rods are placed side by side and $7 + 7$ is written and discussed as being equal to 14. A one rod is placed on the end of a seven rod, increasing the sum to 15 (adding on 1 takes you to the next number). The seven and one rods are exchanged for an eight rod and the addition $7 + 8 = 15$ is discussed:

$(2 + 2) + 1 = 2 + 3 = 5$
$(3 + 3) + 1 = 3 + 4 = 7$
$(3 + 3) - 1 = 3 + 2 = 5$
$(4 + 4) + 1 = 4 + 5 = 9$
$(4 + 4) - 1 = 4 + 3 = 7$
$(5 + 5) + 1 = 5 + 6 = 11$
$(5 + 5) - 1 = 5 + 4 = 9$, etc.

This gives seven facts for the doubles and 12 facts for doubles ±1. The task is down to 30 facts, half of which are commutative, so there are 15 different facts to go.

**Number bonds for 10**

These facts are extensible facts, that is, they can have significant uses in other situations to solve other problems. They are therefore important facts to learn.

There are a variety of concrete images which can be used to illustrate the number bonds to 10.

- Cuisennaire rods (Figure 5.3) give a colourful image of the linear relationship.

- A pile of poker chips (good because they are substantially thick) can be used to show one pile growing as the other decreases as chips are transferred from one pile to the other.

- The number bonds can be written graphically (Figure 5.4).

Whatever materials the child handles, you must make sure that the digits are presented with each manipulative aid.

Although this section collects together the number bonds for 10, only $6 + 4$, $4 + 6$, $7 + 3$ and $3 + 7$ are 'new' facts..., so, 26 to go.

**Number bonds for 9**

These follow on from the number bonds for 10. They are important as part of the strategy for the $9 \times$ table facts. The child has to see that 9 is one less than 10, so the two sets of number bonds need to be compared and the consistent relationship emphasised.

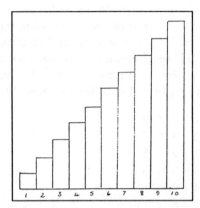

**Figure 5.3**   Cuisenaire rods

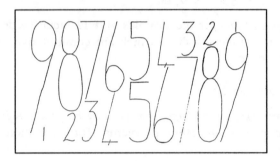

**Figure 5.4**

### Adding on 9

This also follows on from the equivalent 10 facts. They are also useful as an introduction to estimation. The child is learning again that 10 is one more than 9 and that 9 is one less than 10.

The child can practise the addition with coins or base-ten blocks, comparing adding ten with adding nine, looking at adding 9 by adding 10 then subtracting 1, or using the added number to provide 1 to make the 9 up to 10 (and the added number one less), e.g. $9 + 6 = 10 + 6 - 1$ or $9 + 6 = (9 + 1) + (6 - 1)$.

These two groups of nine facts add 12 more facts, leaving 14 to go.

### Sharing doubles

$n + n$ is the same as $(n - 1) + (n + 1)$. There are six of these facts:

3 + 5 and 5 + 3 are the same as $4 + 4 = 8$.

5 + 7 and 7 + 5 are the same as $6 + 6 = 12$.

8 + 6 and 6 + 8 are the same as $7 + 7 = 14$.

(The others are: $2 + 4$ & $4 + 2$; $4 + 6$ & $6 + 4$; $7 + 9$ & $9 + 7$.)

Again these facts can be experienced by moving counters between two initially equal piles. The strategy is an example of the conservation of number and is worth inclusion for learning this alone.

There are eight facts to go. The commutative property reduces this to four: $8 + 3$, $8 + 4$, $8 + 5$, $7 + 4$.

Adding onto 8 can be achieved via 10, e.g. $8 + 5$ becomes $(8 + 2) + 3$. $7 + 4$ can be seen as one more than the number bond $7 + 3$.

**Summary**

Some of the facts described in this chapter fall into more than one strategy group. As flexibility is important, this gives the child some choice of method. Shading squares for families of strategies in fact emphasises the pattern of each relationship.

In each strategy there is ample scope to have the child use concrete manipulative materials. These materials must be used *and* used in conjunction with showing the child the written numbers. The child has to learn to progress from the concrete to the symbolic and the process has to be multisensory. Again, with each strategy, the child must practise using the digits. Kirkby (1989, 1992, 1993; see Appendix) has some useful games to add variety and motivation to the practice (and may help to reduce the frequency of transpositions, such as 42 for 24).

# Subtraction Facts

When writing and talking about the addition facts, you must use more than one format, for example, $4 + 6 = 10$ can be phrased as:

- What is 4 add 6?

- What adds on to 4 to make 10?

- Can you find the 'right' number to fit into the box:

$4 + 6 = \square$ $\qquad$ $4 + \square = 10$ $\qquad$ $\square + 6 = 10$ ?

The latter two examples are leading the child to see subtraction as 'adding on'. $4 + 6 = \square$ is a straight addition fact. The child is, however, learning that 10 can be split into two constituent parts, in this case 4 and 6. With $4 + \square = 10$ and $\square + 6 = 10$ the child still has to know that we are looking at two parts, but he now knows the total and only one of the parts. We are changing the frame of reference, not the knowledge.

Further examples and the introduction of the vocabulary of subtraction (minus, subtract, $-$, etc.) should lead the child to transfer his addition facts into subtraction facts. The idea of a total or sum and two parts or addends will be used in 'harder' subtraction problems in the next chapter.

addends will be used in 'harder' subtraction problems in the next chapter.

The child needs to learn that addition and subtraction are variations of the same process (Ashcroft and Chinn, 1992). The ideas above provide the framework which you can use and develop into an instructional format.

## Extension

Ashcroft and Chinn (1992) advocate the use of patterns and sequences. For example, addition facts can be extended to the sequence/pattern

$$4 + \phantom{0}7 = 11 \qquad \phantom{0}4 + 7 = 11$$
$$4 + 17 = 21 \qquad 14 + 7 = 21$$
$$4 + 27 = 31 \qquad 24 + 7 = 31$$
$$4 + 37 = 41 \qquad 34 + 7 = 41$$
$$4 + 47 = 51 \qquad 44 + 7 = 51 \text{, etc.}$$

which shows the consistent contribution of $4 + 7$ to a sequence of sums. The dyslexic child often needs the aspects of this pattern (and similar patterns) pointing out to him. In doing this, you are also leading the child towards addition sums, where he will be using the addition facts and, hopefully, reinforcing his knowledge of these facts.

# Chapter 6
# Times Tables

## Introduction

Whenever there is a back-to-basics movement in education, the issue of learning times tables (and other basic facts) arises. To a large extent this argument is irrelevant for dyslexics. In our combined experience of over 20 years of teaching mathematics to dyslexics, we have found that the rote learning of times tables is a frustrating exercise for both learner and teacher (see also Miles, 1983; Pritchard et al., 1989).

We believe that there is an effective alternative solution to this problem. Although we suggest an effective rote learning technique, we believe that strategies based on patterns and the interrelationships of numbers are effective in learning how to work out times-table facts. These strategies give the learner routes to an answer, as opposed to him or her relying on memory which gives no possibilty of obtaining a correct answer when he or she forgets the fact. Again, our experience is that many children already use strategies which they have devised for themselves, though often these strategies are neither consistent nor organised mathematically.

## Rote Learning with Tape Recorders

### Use of music

There are tapes of times tables set to music. The rhythm and the tune help some to learn the tables, but in our experience, only a few.

### The ARROW technique

The learner can use the ARROW technique (Lane and Chinn, 1986; Lane, 1990), as described in Chapter 4. This is a multisensory method using the learner's own voice recorded on tape. Tape recorders with a review button are easiest to use.

1. The child copies out the table facts he wishes to learn.

2. He records them onto tape, in groups of about four facts at a time, leaving a three to five second gap between each fact.

3. He puts on headphones and listens to the first fact. He stops the tape.

4. He says the fact and writes it. He rewinds the tape back to the start of the fact.

5. He listens again to the fact. He repeats steps 4 and 5 three or four more times.

6. He repeats steps 3, 4 and 5 with the next fact.

The learner should experiment within this basic structure to find which multisensory procedure is the most effective. The listening frequently encourages sub-vocalising, which also reinforces learning. This can be a very effective method for many people, but not for all.

The process should be repeated several days in a row for the same set of facts. The learner will probably find that five to ten facts per session are enough, but success has a great motivating effect, so more may be possible.

## Learning by Understanding

There are many advantages in learning times-table facts by understanding. The methods we advocate provide memory 'hooks' on which to hang several connected facts and some of them are introductions to procedures used later on in mathematics, such as estimation. The strategies suggested here encourage the learner to look for patterns and interrelationships between numbers; they help develop a facility with numbers.

It is our experience that the basic structure for the strategy approach uses the times-table square, even though initial work is with separate tables. The square gives an overview of the task and can be used to illustrate gains in an encouraging way.

There are 121 facts in the table square (Figure 6.1). The size of this task can be reduced quite quickly and easily. This progress can be readily shown to the learner and contrasts with the normal approach of, 'Which tables do you know?'.

You (the teacher) should ask the child to look at the table with you, to see several helpful things.

| × | 0 | 1 | 2 | 3 | 4 | 5 | 6 | 7 | 8 | 9 | 10 |
|---|---|---|---|---|---|---|---|---|---|---|---|
| 0 | 0 | 0 | 0 | 0 | 0 | 0 | 0 | 0 | 0 | 0 | 0 |
| 1 | 0 | 1 | 2 | 3 | 4 | 5 | 6 | 7 | 8 | 9 | 10 |
| 2 | 0 | 2 | 4 | 6 | 8 | 10 | 12 | 14 | 16 | 18 | 20 |
| 3 | 0 | 3 | 6 | 9 | 12 | 15 | 18 | 21 | 24 | 27 | 30 |
| 4 | 0 | 4 | 8 | 12 | 16 | 20 | 24 | 28 | 32 | 36 | 40 |
| 5 | 0 | 5 | 10 | 15 | 20 | 25 | 30 | 35 | 40 | 45 | 50 |
| 6 | 0 | 6 | 12 | 18 | 24 | 30 | 36 | 42 | 48 | 54 | 60 |
| 7 | 0 | 7 | 14 | 21 | 28 | 35 | 42 | 49 | 56 | 63 | 70 |
| 8 | 0 | 8 | 16 | 24 | 32 | 40 | 48 | 56 | 64 | 72 | 80 |
| 9 | 0 | 9 | 18 | 27 | 36 | 45 | 54 | 63 | 72 | 81 | 90 |
| 10 | 0 | 10 | 20 | 30 | 40 | 50 | 60 | 70 | 80 | 90 | 100 |

**Figure 6.1** The times-table square

## Patterns

There are patterns, e.g. the column and row for the 10-times facts is 10 20 30 40 50 60 70 80 90 100, the numbers from 1 to 10 with an extra digit, a 0, at the end (see also place value). If information can be seen to be in patterns or if it can be organised in patterns, it is easier to learn. There is also a sound pattern for the 10-times facts which links to the numbers one to nine: ten, twenty, thirty, forty, fifty, sixty, seventy, eighty, ninety – one of us (S.C.) uses 'tenty' as well as one hundred to reinforce the pattern, to emphasise the place-value need for a special word for 100 and to refer to when in subtraction a hundred is renamed as ten lots of ten – 'tenty'. It's also fun.

There are other patterns in the square which the child can look at later. At this stage you are introducing an idea. You must use your professional judgement to see how far you can go at this stage without becoming counter-productive.

## Numbers which do not appear

Not all the numbers between 0 and 100 appear, e.g. 43. This does not mean they are not important, just less used in this area of work.

## Limiting the task

The numbers have a lowest value of 0, and a highest value of 100. So the child has some limits for the task and the task can be made to appear possible and, with a little understanding of how numbers relate to each other, even more possible.

Remember that each time the child learns a set of facts, the task gets smaller. Furthermore, when he learns a fact from say the 5-times table, e.g. $5 \times 7 = 35$, he also learns $7 \times 5 = 35$, two facts for the price of one. This commutative property needs to be introduced quite early in the work.

You will note that the square does not include 11 times or 12 times. This is quite deliberate. Both can be taught, if deemed necessary, by strategies based on $11 = 10 + 1$ and $12 = 10 + 2$.

## The Order in which to Learn the Facts

It seems sensible to learn first the facts which lead to the quickest gains and therefore encourage confidence. You may wish to change the order given in Table 6.1, but we suggest that the first three remain set as shown. In our experience, the order of learning the 5-times and 9-times tables could be interchanged.

**Table 6.1** Times-table learning

| Times table | Number of facts left to learn |
|:-----------:|:-----------------------------:|
| 0's | 100 |
| 1's | 81 |
| 10's | 64 |
| 2's | 49 |
| 5's | 36 |
| 9's | 25 |

So by the time the child has learnt the times tables listed in Table 6.1, he has reduced his task from 121 facts to learn down to 25. These first 96 facts are the easiest to learn and you can quickly demonstrate how the child can start to make rapid gains.

### Quick check backs

Constant reviews are important. You are dealing with severe short- and long-term memory deficits. It is beneficial to revise and review material with the child quite often and, as with all skills, a lack of practice will reduce the skill level. This is especially so with dyslexics. We maintain that learning-check charts with headings 'Taught, Revised, Learnt' should also have a fourth column for use with dyslexics, 'Forgotten'.

## The Commutative Property

The commutative property is expressed algebraically as:

$$a \times b = b \times a$$

It can be introduced to a child as a way of getting double value for most of the times-table facts that he learns (not the squares).

One of the models or pictures for 'times' is area. Squared paper is useful for this model. To illustrate the commutative property a learner can draw a rectangle of $4 \times 10$, oriented to have the side of 10 units horizontal, then he can draw a second rectangle, $10 \times 4$, with the side of 10 units vertical. These areas can represent rooms or carpets. If it is not obvious that the two areas are the same, then the learner can count the squares or, if prone to miscounting, cut out the two rectangles and place them on top of one another to show they are the same size (Figure 6.2).

Another illustration of the same property can be achieved with Cuisenaire rods. So for $3 \times 5$ and $5 \times 3$, three five rods (yellows) can be put down to make a rectangle and then five three rods (light green) can be placed next to them to show that $3 \times 5$ and $5 \times 3$ cover the same area (and that three lots of five and five lots of three are the same) (Figure 6.3).

Another effective demonstration which focuses on the 'lots of' version of 'times' is to use counters in rows and columns. This additional 'picture' reinforces and develops further understanding of the concept of multiplication. For example, twelve counters can be placed down as three rows of four or as four rows of three (Figure 6.4).

Each of these methods looks at a different facet of multiplication and each has future currency; this suggests that all three should be used to demonstrate and reinforce the concept. Examples of future currency are using area to provide a picture of multiplications such as $(a + b) (a + 3b)$, and extending $5 \times 8$ from five lots of of eight to six lots of eight.

You have then demonstrated that $4 \times 10$ is exactly the same as $10 \times 4$, that $5 \times 8 = 8 \times 5$, that $3 \times 7 = 7 \times 3$ and so on.

Each fact the child learns can have the order changed round, giving him another fact – free! You may wish to digress to discuss squares, such as $4 \times 4$ – judge the readiness of the class.

## Learning the Table Square

## Zero: 0

Zero is an important concept, so time should be spent establishing that the child has some understanding of zero; zero, nought, nothing – as ever the language should be varied.

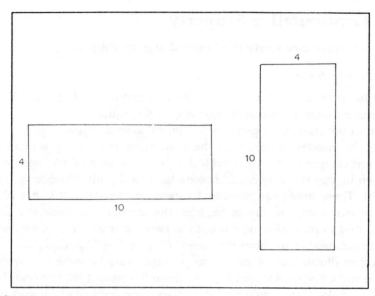

**Figure 6.2** Using area

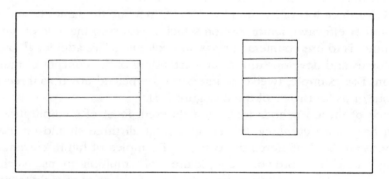

**Figure 6.3** Using Cuisenaire rods

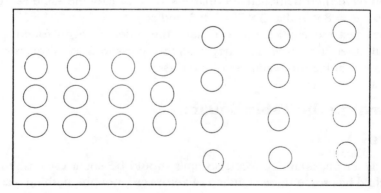

**Figure 6.4** Using counters

In later numeracy work the child will meet examples like $304 \times 23$ or $406 + 2$, where the process of multiplying a zero, multiplying by zero or dividing into zero is used. You can start by explaining the meaning of $3 \times 0$ and so on: $3 \times 0$ means:

3 times 0

or three lots of 0 giving the answer 0.

$0 \times 3$ is the same, zero lots of 3 is also zero.

*Two suggested teaching models*

- Talk about having nothing in one pocket, nothing in two pockets and so on.

- Use empty 35 mm film tubes and discuss how much in one empty tube, two empty tubes and so on.

The child should then realise that any number times 0 equals 0 and 0 times any number equals 0. So

$$1 \times 0 = 0 \quad \text{and} \quad 0 \times 1 = 0$$

$$2 \times 0 = 0 \qquad 0 \times 2 = 0$$

$$3 \times 0 = 0 \qquad 0 \times 3 = 0$$

Children like massive examples such as a million lots of zero or zero lots of a million – it impresses much more than zero lots of two even if the result is the same!

Now you can tell the child to look at the table square.

You will see a row of 0's across the top, and a column of 0's down the left hand side. You have just learnt your first 21 facts.

*Progress check*

If you want the child to keep a check on his progress use the table square in Figure 6.1. Copy one and hand it to the child to act as his record of progress. Tell him to shade in all the zero facts – the top row and the first column. (You will probably find the child needs a second table square to keep as a 'clean' copy.)

# One: 1

One is the basic unit: $4 \times 1$ means:

4 times 1

or 4 lots of 1 gives the answer 4.

$1 \times 4$ is the same.

Any number times 1 equals that number.

1 times any number equals that number.

Counters are quite a good manipulative aid for demonstration (they can also be used on an overhead projector), or for the child to use to understand 'one lot of' or '$n$ lots of'. Money can also be introduced here in the form of pennies. So $7 \times 1 = 7$ (seven lots of one) and $1 \times 6 = 6$ (one lot of six) and so on.

The concept you are introducing here is summed up by the equations:

$n \times 1 = n$ and $1 \times n = n$

Again tell the child to look back at the table square and see that the 1-times table facts appear twice, first written across, second row down; then written down, second column in.

$$1 \times \phantom{0}0 = \phantom{0}0$$
$$1 \times \phantom{0}1 = \phantom{0}1$$
$$1 \times \phantom{0}2 = \phantom{0}2$$
$$1 \times \phantom{0}3 = \phantom{0}3$$
$$1 \times \phantom{0}4 = \phantom{0}4$$
$$1 \times \phantom{0}5 = \phantom{0}5$$
$$1 \times \phantom{0}6 = \phantom{0}6$$
$$1 \times \phantom{0}7 = \phantom{0}7$$
$$1 \times \phantom{0}8 = \phantom{0}8$$
$$1 \times \phantom{0}9 = \phantom{0}9$$
$$1 \times 10 = 10$$

Again explain and demonstrate the important fact that the number you multiply by 1 does not change in value (the use of the phrase 'in value' could be considered pedantic, but it is important not to teach information which has to be 'unlearned' at a later date, e.g. in fractions). When 1 multiplies a number it leaves the number with the same value as it had before.

$$0 \times 1 = \phantom{0}0$$
$$1 \times 1 = \phantom{0}1$$
$$2 \times 1 = \phantom{0}2$$
$$3 \times 1 = \phantom{0}3$$
$$\cdot$$
$$\cdot$$
$$\cdot$$
$$10 \times 1 = 10$$

The child has now learnt 19 new facts (he had already learnt $0 \times 1$ and $1 \times 0$), making a total so far of 40 out of 121 – almost a third.

*Progress check*

The child can now shade in the one facts. He shades in the second row and the second column. These are the numbers 1 to 10 across and down.

# Ten: 10

1, 2, 3, 4, 5, 6, 7, 8, 9 are single digits. 10 has two digits, a 1 followed by a 0. The 0 means no units, and the 1 means 1 ten. Hopefully the child has retained earlier work on place value from Chapter 4. A moment's re-inforcement will check this.

Ten is a key number in this chapter. The 10-times table facts will be extended to teach the child how to work out the 5-times facts and the 9-times facts. Thus it is well worth reviewing the child's understanding of 10 and place value.

So explain that 20 has a 0 for 0 units and a 2 for 2 tens. $2 \times 10$ means:

2 times 10 equals 20

2 lots of 10 are 20.

There is an easy pattern to show:

| A | B | B |
|---|---|---|
| $1 \times 10 =$ | 1 | 0 |
| $2 \times 10 =$ | 2 | 0 |
| $3 \times 10 =$ | 3 | 0 |
| $4 \times 10 =$ | 4 | 0 |
| $5 \times 10 =$ | 5 | 0 |
| $6 \times 10 =$ | 6 | 0 |
| $7 \times 10 =$ | 7 | 0 |
| $8 \times 10 =$ | 8 | 0 |
| $9 \times 10 =$ | 9 | 0 |
| $10 \times 10 =$ | 10 | 0 |

- The numbers under A are the first ten units.

- The numbers under BB are the first ten tens.

Get the child to listen to the pattern as he says the 10-times table and sees the connection: e.g.

six tens are sixty,

nine tens are ninety.

Even two tens are twenty gives a two-letter clue. We find that a brief digression to 'twoty', 'threety' and 'fivety' reinforces rather than confuses.

This pattern can be practised with trading money, always remembering to have the child say as he trades one 1p coin for one 10p coin, 'one times ten is ten'. He then trades two 1p coins for two 10p coins, and says 'two times ten is twenty'.

And so on, till he trades $10 \times 10p$ coins for ten 10p coins, and says 'ten times ten is tenty'; there is no such word of course and a special word is used instead – hundred. A hundred, 100, has three digits, the only number with three digits in the table square. A hundred pence has its own coin, a pound. So $10 \times 10p = 100p = 1$ pound.

There are other ways to practise the units/tens relationship.

- Single cocktail sticks, and bundles of ten cocktail sticks:

    1 stick $\times 10$ = 1  bundle  = 10

    2 sticks $\times 10$ = 2  bundles = 20

    3 sticks $\times 10$ = 3  bundles = 30;

    each time 'ten times bigger' means exchanging a ten-stick bundle for a single stick.

- Cuisenaire rods:

    1 unit  $\times 10$ = 1  of ten strips = 10

    3 units $\times 10$ = 3   of ten strips = 30

    and so on (Figure 6.5).

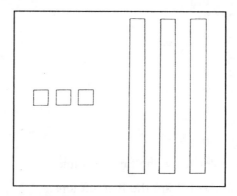

**Figure 6.5**

- Base ten (Dienes) blocks or a metre rule can be used to add to the development of the idea of the 10-times table. A useful illustration from the child's (probable) experience is the idea of change machines, one giving 1p coins and one giving 10p coins and pressing, for example, the '4' button on each; one gives 4p, the other gives 40p.

Remember that some materials are proportional in size to their value, e.g. Cuisenaire rods; some are proportional in number, e.g. bundles of sticks;

some are proportional by volume, e.g. base-ten blocks; some are proportional by length, e.g. a metre rule; some are representative of value, e.g. 1p and 10p coins. Using a mixture of these *and the numbers themselves* ensures development from concrete to symbolic understanding.

Some 'everyday' examples may be used to provide reinforcement:

- How many legs on ten cows?

- How many wheels on ten bikes?

- How many pence in ten 5p coins?

- How many legs on ten spiders?

- How many sides on ten 50p coins?

*Progress check*

If the child thinks that he has learnt the 10-times facts then he can shade in the end column and the bottom row of his table square, the 10-times facts. Filling in the tens' column and the tens' row should remind the child that for each times fact he can write the numbers in either order, so, for example, $2 \times 10 = 10 \times 2$. This means that, if he remembers that $10 \times 3 = 30$, then he knows $3 \times 10 = 30$, one fact from the 3-times table and one fact from the 10-times table – two for the price of one! The commutative property should be reinforced frequently.

So far the child has learnt 57 facts, almost half. He has 64 to learn.

# Two: 2

First, as for each number, the lessons should look at the concept of the number and its interrelationships with other numbers. There can be some demonstrations and discussions and some information on 2, such as:

- Two is one more than one.

- It is twice as big as one.

- It is an even number.

- Even numbers are numbers that share into two equal parts.

  *Example:*

  8 divides (shares) into two lots of 4:

  $8 \div 2 = 4$ or $8 = 4 + 4$.

  20 divides into two lots of 10:

  $20 \div 2 = 10$ or $20 = 10 + 10$.

Each child can try equal sharing with a random pile of pennies, sharing them out, one at a time, into two piles. If the two piles are equal, then he started with an *even* number. If there is one penny left over, then he started with an *odd* number.

- Even numbers from 1 to 10 are 2, 4, 6, 8, 10.

- Odd numbers from 1 to 10 are 1, 3, 5, 7, 9.

A useful extra fact (generalisation) here is that any even number ends in 2, 4, 6, 8 or 0, and any odd number ends in 1, 3, 5, 7 or 9.

Some review/revision questions can be used, such as:

- Which of these numbers is even? 2341, 4522, 57399, 34, 70986, 11112, 335792.

- Which of them divide evenly by two?

- If the pattern for even numbers is:

      2   4   6   8   10
     12  14  16  18  20
     22  24  26  28  30

continue the pattern to 102.

## The 2-times table

<table>
<tr><td>$1 \times 2 = 2$</td><td>*Notice:*</td></tr>
<tr><td>$2 \times 2 = 4$</td><td>1. The end number pattern repeats 2, 4, 6,</td></tr>
<tr><td>$3 \times 2 = 6$</td><td>   8, 0.</td></tr>
<tr><td>$4 \times 2 = 8$</td><td></td></tr>
<tr><td>$5 \times 2 = 10$</td><td>2. The answers are the same as in the</td></tr>
<tr><td>$6 \times 2 = 12$</td><td>   even number table the child did earlier.</td></tr>
<tr><td>$7 \times 2 = 14$</td><td></td></tr>
<tr><td>$8 \times 2 = 16$</td><td></td></tr>
<tr><td>$9 \times 2 = 18$</td><td></td></tr>
<tr><td>$10 \times 2 = 20$</td><td></td></tr>
</table>

The first four facts can be learnt as a chant:

Two, four, six, eight, who(m) do we appreciate?

This chant brings the child to almost half-way in learning the 2-times table.

Often it is useful to have *reference points* in calculations. The child already has a start reference point, $1 \times 2 = 2$, and an end reference point, $10 \times 2 = 20$. The middle reference point has its value on the child's hands – two hands, each with five fingers, two lots of five fingers, ten fingers, $2 \times 5 = 10$ or $5 \times 2 = 10$. It also is illustrated by $5 \times 2p = 10p$, a trading operation, where five 2p coins are traded for one 10p coin. So $5 \times 2 = 10$ is the middle reference point on which to build the remaining facts $6 \times 2$ to $10 \times 2$.

The answers for $6 \times 2$ to $9 \times 2$ have the same last digits as the first four facts, 12, 14, 16, 18 – the child needs to be shown the pattern. They have the same digit pattern because $6 \times 2$ is one more 2 than $5 \times 2$ and $7 \times 2$ is two more 2's than $5 \times 2$, etc. and because $5 \times 2$ has 0 in its units digit column. This is the first use of the strategy of a middle reference point, which in this case combines with the strategy of breaking down numbers to build up on a known fact.

So if the child can remember the reference value $5 \times 2 = 10$, he can quickly work out, say, $8 \times 2$. 8 is $5 + 3$, so $8 \times 2$ is five lots of 2 plus three lots of 2, so $8 \times 2 = (5 \times 2) + (3 \times 2) = 10 + 6 = 16$.

There are three useful and regularly occurring strategies here:

1. Breaking down a number, e.g. 8 into 5 and 3, so that earlier facts are used and extended.

2. The use of a reference point in the middle of the task. A child will claim to 'know' the 2-times table. When asked for $7 \times 2$ he begins at 2 and works up 2, 4, 6, 8, 10, 12, 14. A middle reference point means that the child can start at 10.

3. The use of 'lots of' for times leads to six lots of 2 being seen as one more lot (of 2) than five lots of 2.

*Strategies need practice and reinforcement*

Some practical work can be built around coins and trading, using a 10p coin for tens and 2p coins for two. The learner trades five lots of 2p for a 10p coin to reinforce the middle reference point and the repeating 2, 4, 6, 8 pattern. An example with $8 \times 2$ is to take eight 2p coins, take out five of these and trade them for a 10p coin. This leaves one 10p coin and three 2p coins, which combine as 10 and $3 \times 2$ to make 16.

# Five: 5

As with all the times tables, the first step is to establish a basic understanding of the number, in this case 5.

## Some information about 5

- The key fact is that five is half-way from zero to ten. The learner can be reminded how five was used as a half-way reference point in the 2-times table, i.e. five is half of ten.

- Ten divided by two is five. It can be written in numbers as: $10 \div 2 = 5$.

- Five is an odd number.

- Five can look like 5 or lllll or V or 10/2 or $10 \div 2$.

## The 5-times table

| | |
|---|---|
| $1 \times 5 =$ | 5 |
| $2 \times 5 =$ | 10 |
| $3 \times 5 =$ | 15 |
| $4 \times 5 =$ | 20 |
| $5 \times 5 =$ | 25 |
| $6 \times 5 =$ | 30 |
| $7 \times 5 =$ | 35 |
| $8 \times 5 =$ | 40 |
| $9 \times 5 =$ | 45 |
| $10 \times 5 =$ | 50 |

*Notice:*

1. The child knows the start reference point $1 \times 5 = 5$, and the end reference point $10 \times 5 = 50$.

2. There is a pattern in the last 5 digits: 5, 0, 5, 0, 5, 0, 5, 0, 5, 0.

3. This means another pattern: an (odd number times five) gives an answer which ends in 5 and an (even number times five) gives an answer which ends in 0.

It is useful to set up a comparison of the 10- and 5-times tables by writing the answers side by side. Looking at the answers illustrates the relationship between them, i.e. each 5-times answer is half of each 10-times answer, e.g. $6 \times 5 = 30$ and $6 \times 10 = 60$, and 30 is half of 60. It is possible to work out the fives by taking the tens and halving the answers. So, for $8 \times 5$, $8 \times 10 = 80$ and half of 80 is 40. As a check, 8 is even, so the answer ends in 0. Again, for $5 \times 5$: $5 \times 10 = 50$ and half of 50 is 25. As a check, 5 is odd, so the answer ends in 5.

This strategy of looking at the last digit helps reinforce the child's attention on reviewing an answer and its validity.

## Some practical work

The learner can practise halving tens by trading 10p and 5p coins; for each 10p trade one 5p. Each time you must help the child rehearse the process:

Seven times five. Start at seven times ten. Half of seventy is thirty plus five, that is thirtyfive. Seven was odd. The answer ends in a five. That checks.

This can be reinforced by taking seven 5p coins and explaining that they are worth half as much as seven 10p coins.

If the child has difficulty in dividing 30, 50, 70 and 90 by 2, remind the child how to break numbers down, e.g. 50 is $40 + 10$. Halve 40 (answer 20) and halve 10 (answer 5), so that $50 \div 2 = 25$.

Again you may have to remind the child how sometimes it is easier to use two small, quick steps than to struggle with one difficult step.

Other materials may be used to reinforce this relationship between five and ten; these include Cuisenaire rods, 5p and 10p coins and 35 mm film tubes with 5 or 10 items inside. This last material emphasises the 'lots of' aspect of multiplication, used when extending knowledge of, say five 'lots of' to six or seven 'lots of'.

As before, the target is for the learner to be able to recall a 5-times table fact from memory or work out an answer quickly. Starting from $1 \times 5$ and counting up to the required answer is not the target. When the learner can remember or work out the 5-times facts, then he can shade in the five row and column on his table square. The times-table task is reduced to 36 facts.

# Nine: 9

There is an easy method to work out the 9-times facts using fingers. If we were being rigidly principled, we might not mention a method which is radically different from the other methods and strategies mentioned in this book. However, working with dyslexics can make you very pragmatic and eclectic, on the basis that the gains in the child's self-confidence may outweigh any doubts about the academic validity of a particular technique.

So, if you want to know the answer to $4 \times 9$, for example, put the fingers of both hands down on a surface and tuck back the fourth (4) finger from the left (Figure 6.6). The answer lies each side of this fourth finger, the tens to the left, three fingers means 30, and the units to the right, six fingers, giving an answer of 36.

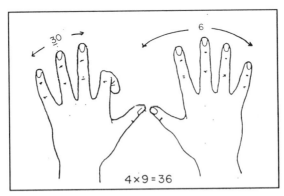

**Figure 6.6**

However, we prefer a strategy with potential for further use. Therefore, the strategy we advocate is based on estimation, the particularly useful estimation of ten for nine, and the subsequent refinement of this estimation.

The first step is to establish the principle of the method, that is that nine is one less than ten. This is helped by examining nine.

- Nine is nine units.

- Nine is one less than ten.

- $9 = 10 - 1$ and $10 = 9 + 1$.

The closeness in value of nine and ten can be demonstrated by showing the child a pile of ten 1p coins and asking him to say, without counting them, if there are nine or ten. It does not matter which the child guesses. It is the uncertainty that is important; the nearness of nine and ten makes it hard to give an answer with certainty. The demonstration can move on to Cuisenaire rods. A ten rod (orange) and a nine rod (blue) are placed side by side. A one rod (white) is added to the nine rod to show that the difference is one. This is presented in numerals as

$$9 + 1 = 10 \qquad\qquad 10 - 1 = 9.$$

This demonstration is now extended to show how to estimate and refine from the 10-times table to the 9-times table.

Two nine rods are placed on a flat surface. Two ten rods are placed alongside and two whites are added to the nine rods to show that the difference in value is two. The process is repeated to develop the pattern that $n$ nine rods are $n$ ones less than $n$ ten rods. In numbers:

$$2 \times 10 = 20 \qquad 20 - 2 = 18 \qquad 2 \times 9 = 18$$

$$3 \times 10 = 30 \qquad 30 - 3 = 27 \qquad 3 \times 9 = 27$$

$$4 \times 10 = 40 \qquad 40 - 4 = 36 \qquad 4 \times 9 = 36.$$

Thus any 9-times fact can be worked out from a 10-times fact, for example, $6 \times 9$ is worked out as:

$$6 \times 10 = 60 \qquad 60 - 6 = 54 \qquad 6 \times 9 = 54.$$

This is verbalised as

> Six times nine is six less than six times ten. Six times ten is sixty, so six times nine must be fifty something.

The 'something', the unit digit, can be found by subtracting 6 from 60, or 6 from 10, using number bonds for 10. It can be found by counting backwards from 60, though this is a very difficult task for some dyslexics, or a further pattern can be used:

$$1 \times 9 = \phantom{0}9$$
$$2 \times 9 = 18$$
$$3 \times 9 = 27$$

$4 \times 9 = 36$
$5 \times 9 = 45$
$6 \times 9 = 54$
$7 \times 9 = 63$
$8 \times 9 = 72$
$9 \times 9 = 81$
$10 \times 9 = 90$

*Notice:*
The units column digits go from 9 to 0, whilst the tens column digits go from 0 to 9. This results in the sum of the two digits in each answer always being nine, e.g. for 63, $6 + 3 = 9$.

So the child can work through the following process for, say, $4 \times 9$.

$4 \times 10 = 40$;

$4 \times 9$ is smaller and must be 'thirty something';

the 'something' must be the number which adds on to 3 to make 9, that is 6. So the answer is 36. For $6 \times 9$, again

$6 \times 10 = 60$

$6 \times 9 = 5\square$

$5 + \square = 9$

$\square = 4$ so        $6 \times 9 = 54$

The child may think that this is a long process, but with regular practice it becomes quicker. Also, as the child becomes more adept, he starts to short-circuit the process and use it to top off a half-known answer. In other words, the strategy provides a memory hook for the child so that he is not left floundering when faced with an 'impossible' question.

When the child has grasped this strategy, he may shade in the 9-times column and row. He now has 25 facts left to attack.

# Four: 4

You should give an overview of the properties of four, relating four to other numbers. The most important of these relationships are:

- That $4 = 2 \times 2$.

- Four is twice two.

- Four is four units, 4, IV, 1111.

- Four is two times two.

This last relationship is the basis of the method advocated for the 4-times table. The method is building on knowledge the child has already learnt and makes use of the interrelationships of numbers. The child is taught to double the 2-times table. We have found that effective memory triggers have been to call this the 'tutu' method or the 'double-double' method. You have to establish the strategy using methods such as 2p coins, set up to show the 2-times table alongside the 4-times table, e.g.

$2 \times 2$ compared with $2 \times 4$

$3 \times 2$ compared with $3 \times 4$.

The 2-times table is shown with single piles of 2p coins and the 4-times table is shown with double piles of 2p coins. 35 mm film tubes may also be used to reinforce the idea of comparing three lots of 2 with three lots of 4. The child can see 'three lots of' and it should be possible to convince him that he ends up with twice as much from three tubes with 4p in as he does from three tubes with 2p in. (This is a similar strategy to comparing the 5-times and 10-times tables.)

Once the idea of the strategy is established, you can move on to comparing the answers to the 2-times and 4-times tables in the same way that the 5-times and 10-times tables were compared.

| | | |
|---|---|---|
| $1 \times 2 = 2$ | $4 =$ | $1 \times 4$ |
| $2 \times 2 = 4$ | $8 =$ | $2 \times 4$ |
| $3 \times 2 = 6$ | $12 =$ | $3 \times 4$ |
| $4 \times 2 = 8$ | $16 =$ | $4 \times 4$ |
| $5 \times 2 = 10$ | $20 =$ | $5 \times 4$ |
| $6 \times 2 = 12$ | $24 =$ | $6 \times 4$ |
| $7 \times 2 = 14$ | $28 =$ | $7 \times 4$ |
| $8 \times 2 = 16$ | $32 =$ | $8 \times 4$ |
| $9 \times 2 = 18$ | $36 =$ | $9 \times 4$ |
| $10 \times 2 = 20$ | $40 =$ | $10 \times 4$ |

(It's worth reminding the learner that he already knows $0 \times 4$, $1 \times 4$, $2 \times 4$, $5 \times 4$, $9 \times 4$ and $10 \times 4$ from the tables he has learned previously.)

$1 \times 4$ to $5 \times 4$ are achieved by doubling within the known range of the 2-times table, e.g. the learner can manage $4 \times 4$ as $2 \times 4 = 8$ and $2 \times 8 = 16$ and thus $4 \times 4 = 16$. Some practice to reinforce this 'known' pattern may be needed.

$6 \times 4$ and $7 \times 4$ are relatively easy since there is no carrying to complicate the second doubling:

$6 \times 2 = 12$        $12 \times 2 = 24$

$7 \times 2 = 14$        $14 \times 2 = 28$.

The second doubling of $8 \times 4$ and $9 \times 4$ can be done via break-down strategies, using 8 as $5 + 3$ and 9 as $5 + 4$ or $10 - 1$. Alternatively, $9 \times 4$ can be done as $4 \times 9$ from the 9-times table.

It may be good practice for the learner to give you the middle step in practice sessions so that $7 \times 4$ is delivered in two stages: 14 then 28.

When the 4-times facts are shaded in on the table square the learner has just 16 facts to learn. Six of these are commutative, leaving only ten separate facts. It is possible to take these piecemeal, or to teach the 3-times facts as 2-times then add one more, i.e. $2a + a$. (This strategy is also of use to extend $6 \times 5$, via $5 \times 6$ to $6 \times 6$, i.e. $5a + a = 6a$.)

## Six: 6; Seven: 7; Eight: 8

The target has now been lowered to nine facts or six separate facts:

$7 \times 8$, $6 \times 8$, $7 \times 6$, $6 \times 6$, $7 \times 7$ and $8 \times 8$.

These six are often perceived as the hardest to learn, but there are some helpful strategies here, too. As we said above, you can teach $6 \times 6$, $7 \times 6$ and $8 \times 6$ by extending $5 \times 6$, $5 \times 7$ and $5 \times 8$. If you take $6 \times 8$ (and therefore $8 \times 6$) as an example:

- Show, using counters, that $8 \times 5$ (via $8 \times 10$ as revision) is the same as $5 \times 8$.

- Then use film tubes to show that six lots of 8 are one more lot of 8 than five lots of 8.

The film tubes emphasise the move from 'five lots of' to 'six lots of' whilst the contents (8) are seen to be what is added on to the 40. This should help explain the strategy and avoid the child obtaining 46, the most likely error.

This leaves three remaining facts: $6 \times 7$; $7 \times 7$; $8 \times 7$.

The hardest fact is $8 \times 7$. A pattern, which appeals more to adults than to children, is seen if the normal order of presentation is reversed:

5678        $56 = 7 \times 8$.

(This order occurs one other time in the table square with $12 = 3 \times 4$.)

$7 \times 8$ could also be taught by the following sequence;

$8 \times 5 \rightarrow 5 \times 8 \rightarrow 7 = 5 + 2 \rightarrow 7 \times 8 = 5 \times 8 + 2 \times 8 = 40 + 16 = 56$.

$6 \times 7$ and $7 \times 7$ could be taught by similar sequences.

The comparison of $7 \times 7 = 49$ (1 less than 50, which is half a 100) with $10 \times 10 = 100$ is interesting, and makes a useful cutting up exercise with squared paper. This can be extended to build up $7 \times 7$ from $5 \times 5 + 2(5 \times 2) + 2 \times 2$, although $5 \times 7 + 2 \times 7$ is likely to be easier.

Again, you are showing how to build up and break down an answer.

**Final notes**

$6 \times 6$, $7 \times 7$ and $8 \times 8$ are connected to $5 \times 7$, $6 \times 8$ and $7 \times 9$ by

$$a \times a = (a-1)(a+1)+1$$

$$6 \times 6 = (5 \times 7) \times 1; \qquad 6 \times 6 = 36 \qquad 5 \times 7 = 35$$

$$7 \times 7 = (6 \times 8) + 1; \qquad 7 \times 7 = 49 \qquad 6 \times 8 = 48$$

$$8 \times 8 = (7 \times 9) + 1; \qquad 8 \times 8 = 64 \qquad 7 \times 9 = 63.$$

$8 \times 8$ can be explored in terms of powers of 2:

$$8 \times 8 = 8 \times 4 \times 2 = 4 \times 4 \times 2 \times 2 = 16 \times 2 \times 2 = 32 \times 2 = 64.$$

$6 \times 6$ can be explored in terms of three dozen:

$$6 \times 6 = 3 \times 2 \times 6 = 3 \times 12 = 36.$$

In these strategies you are introducing factors, as you did with the tutu method.

## Summary

In this chapter we have introduced the idea of teaching strategies to learn/work out the times-tables facts. We believe that this approach is pragmatic, since few dyslexics can rote-learn this information. It has the added bonus of teaching several useful mathematical processes and concepts, which include: estimation; that number values are interrelated; the strategy of breaking down numbers into convenient and appropriate parts. We hope that a child may, through these strategies, learn to produce quick answers for the times-table facts, whilst having a back-up strategy for those occasions when the mind goes blank. We have also tried to introduce some flexibility in the methods described, ever mindful of our basic premise that all children do not learn in the same way.

# Chapter 7
# Computational Procedures for Addition and Subtraction

## Introduction

The child's knowledge of basic facts concerning addition and subtraction can now be extended to longer computations. Good teaching will always help a dyslexic, at least to reduce learned difficulties (rather than learning difficulties), but you still need to understand and adjust to your pupil to maximise the chances of effective learning (Miles and Miles, 1992).

Our experience of dyslexics leads us to think that some apparent deficits occur because procedure appears to have no reference or rationale which makes the knowledge seem relevant or distinguishable. For example, directions which rely solely on 'left' and 'right' instructions are less likely to be remembered than directions which include landmarks. The landmarks make the directions more 'real' and concrete.

Addition and subtraction can be taught by multisensory methods and these methods should achieve a double aim. First, the child has the benefit of input through more than one sense and, second, the child has concrete experiences to which he can relate the abstract symbols called numbers. Thus the child may learn to understand an algorithm rather than just to apply it mechanically. Kennedy (1975) refers to research which supports the seemingly obvious statement that children perform better when using algorithms which they understand. The use of multisensory teaching in mathematics makes this more likely, especcially if the materials are used so as to give concrete meaning to the concept.

There have been, however, some cautionary words. Hart (1990) cautions that children do not always relate the 'bricks' to the 'sums'. Thus the concrete materials must be accompanied by the written symbols. You must also remember that children do not all have the same cognitive style and therefore you should encourage the use of global overviews, estimates, detailed algorithms, documentation and evaluation (checking), remembering that some of these operations are more related to one end of the learning spectrum than to the other.

# Estimation

Estimates and evaluations should be encouraged as they serve several purposes.

1. Some dyslexics are likely to transpose numbers so that, for example, 39 becomes 93. Estimates and evaluations reinforce the need to check answers (before and after they have been calculated) and help the pupil to see his possible errors.

2. Estimates and evaluations should be used to check results from calculators, where dyslexics are prone to hit the wrong keys (possibly also in the wrong sequence).

3. Estimates are often a real-life mathematics calculation. For example, a driver may only need to know roughly how many litres of petrol he can buy for £10 rather than to have an answer to three decimal places.

4. Estimates can (and should) use less threatening numbers.

# Addition

Work on the computational procedures for addition should be preceded by a review of place value. You need to remember the dyslexic's need for continual reminders and memory refreshers. Overlearning is an important part of any long-term tuition plan and re-establishing the precursors of a new topic reduces the sources of potential failure. An example is:

$$\begin{array}{r} 38 \\ +27 \\ \hline 515 \end{array}$$

The child adds the unit digits to obtain 15, but fails to realise that the 1 represents a 'ten' and should be added into the tens column. Errors such as these are less likely if the child is taught to preview and review the value of his answers. Again, you should be trying to encourage the child to be flexible in his cognitive processes.

The use of concrete materials adds a multisensory dimension to the teaching. You need to keep in your mind the level of abstraction of the materials you are using and to remember to link the concrete to the symbols.

### A developmental programme for teaching addition

The programme is illustrated by the problem 458 + 376.

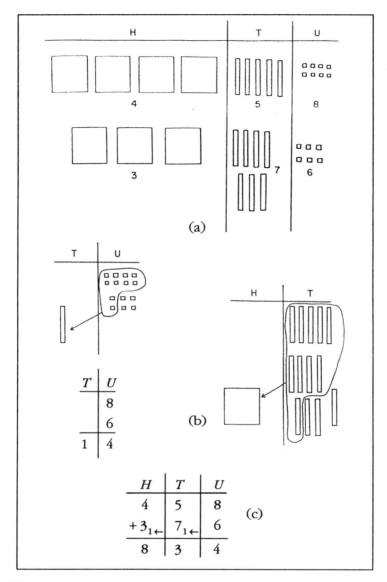

**Figure 7.1**

*Stage 1*

Set the numbers up on a place-value board in base-10 blocks (Figure 7.1a). Tell the child to add (combine/put together) the unit blocks $(8 + 6)$, which gives him 14 unit blocks. You can then discuss this, looking at 14 as four units and one ten. The ten unit blocks can be traded for one 10 block. This is also shown in symbols, so the child relates the written algorithm to the blocks (Figure 7.1b).

Then tell the child to add the 10 blocks $(5 + 7 + 1)$. Encourage the same type of discussion, i.e. the child has 13 ten blocks, which should be viewed as 100 and 30, i.e. one 100 and three 10's. The ten 10 blocks are traded for one 100 block and the operation is written in symbols (digits) so that the child relates the written algorithm to the concrete manipulative aids (Figure 7.1c).

Finally, the hundred column is considered. The blocks show $4 + 3 + 1$ in 100 square blocks, giving a total of eight 100 blocks. Then, take the child through the algorithm again, just in symbols, reminding him of the blocks as each place value is added.

### Stage 2

Repeat the process with coins, explaining how a maximum of 9 pennies is allowed in the units column and the consequent need to trade lots of $10 \times 1p$ for $1 \times 10p$ and $10 \times 10p$ for $1 \times 100p$ (£1) (Figure 7.2).

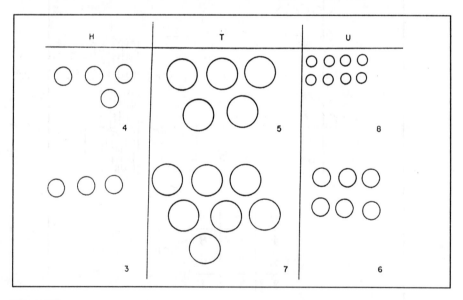

**Figure 7.2**

### Stage 3

Repeat the process with just symbols, but now encourage the child to relate the digit to its place value and discuss the 'carried' number in order to clarify its meaning.

### Estimation

In a problem like the one above $(458 + 376)$ the child can be taught various accuracy levels of estimation. At the simplest level the sum is reduced to the hundred digits (400 + 300). At a more sophisticated level the sum can be presented as 450 + 350 + 30, with the child seeing 458 as approximately 450, but with 8 left over. The 376 is seen as 350 and 25. The 8 from 458 and the 25 from 376 are combined to give an estimate of 30 and the total 450 + 350 + 30 = 830.

The grasshopper (see Chapter 2) may even tackle the complete calculation along these lines, combining convenient parts of the two numbers and mopping up the remainders. For example, he may take 24 from the 458 to make 376 into 400, then add on the 434 which is left. He may take out 350 from 376, 450 from 458 and combine these to make 800, which can be put to one side in short-term memory. Only 8 + 26 is left, which can be added via number bonds for ten as 26 + 4 + 4 = 34. This is added onto the 800 to make 834.

These methods illustrate the advantages of breaking down and building up numbers.

### Column addition

The addition of a column of numbers can be a daunting task. There are two low-stress algorithms (Ashlock, 1982, p. 21) which may help. One (Figure 7.3) is more likely to appeal to inchworms and the other (Figure 7.4) to grasshoppers.

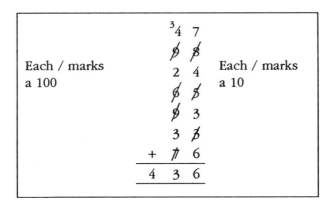

**Figure 7.3** Using tally marks for 10's (and 100's) thereby adding only one-digit sub-sums.

### Mental arithmetic

An extreme inchworm will probably try to visualise a written procedure, e.g. 330 + 97 becomes

330
+ 97
———

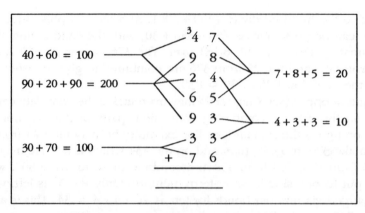

**Figure 7.4** Casting out 10's (or 20's), using again number bonds for 10.

which is added as though on paper, whereas a grasshopper will try to use numbers near to 10, 100 and 1000 or clusters of other numbers which make up 10, 100, 1000, etc. Thus, $330 + 97$ becomes $330 + 100 = 430$, then $430 - 3$ takes the grasshopper to the right answer, 427.

The latter process is usually a lesser strain on short-term memory, and requires less knowledge of basic facts.

# A Developmental Programme for Teaching Subtraction

It may be necessary for you to provide an overview to remind or re-establish the concept and vocabulary of subtraction before teaching specific algorithms. Some examples to which the child can relate, such as change from shopping and/or examples using manipulative aids, are suitable.

You should be trying to establish in the child's mind a clear picture of the component parts of the subtraction. It is usually unnecessary to use the mathematical terms minuend, subtrahend and remainder, but the child needs to understand the consequences of subtraction and be able to relate it to addition.

### Subtraction without regrouping

This is the easiest process and acts as a good introduction as well as re-inforcing the concept of subtraction and the identification of the component parts of the sum. Thus a subtraction such as

$$
\begin{array}{r}
79 \\
-34 \\
\hline
45
\end{array}
$$

may be used to practise the use of manipulative materials such as money or base-ten blocks. Such manipulative work may have to use a place-value board. There is, as ever, a need to teach estimating and to re-emphasise its value as a reducer of errors.

### Subtraction with regrouping: the decomposition method

This method is a relatively recent introduction to teaching and is well illustrated by base-ten blocks (and money). As with so much in mathematics, the work here relies on previous concepts and therefore these concepts may need attention before the main agenda is started. The main review here is to look again at the regrouping of numbers, e.g. 72 is also $60 + 12$ (as spoken in French) or at the renaming (a more descriptive term) of numbers such as 742 to the specific format $600 + 130 + 12$.

Work on renaming three-digit numbers into this format can be investigated and the consequent patterns derived. Examples are:

$$543 = 400 + 130 + 13$$
$$754 = 600 + 140 + 14$$
$$865 = 700 + 150 + 15$$
$$976 = 800 + 160 + 16.$$

The application of this renaming process should lead on to subtraction examples set up on a place-value board with the teacher talking the child through the algorithm. For example:

$$742$$
$$-386$$

The blocks (Figure 7.5a – used first, followed by money) should be moved by the child and the progression should be from base-ten blocks to money, each time writing the numbers as the manipulatives are moved. If the child seems to be understanding the work, then you may take the child to working with just the digits. The child may well need to start with place-value columns drawn on the paper.

Spatial and organisational problems may make the traditional layout too confusing, at least at first, so an intermediate presentation may help. A separate middle line is set up with all the renaming done at one time and before the actual subtraction (Figure 7.5b).

Finally the place-value columns can be removed and the child works on squared or lined paper (Figure 7.5c).

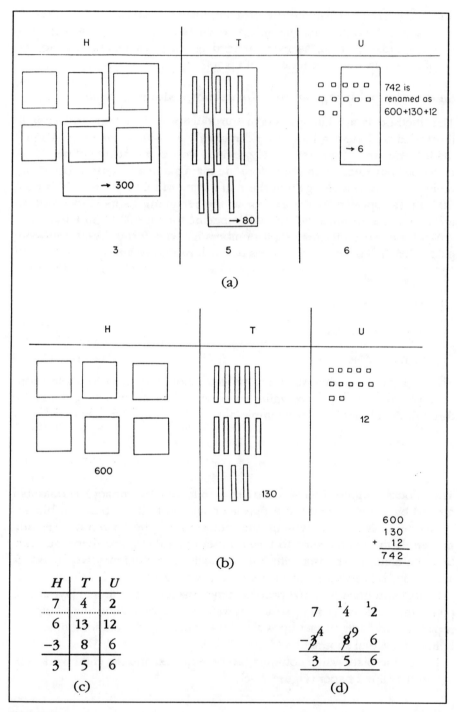

**Figure 7.5**

## The equal-additions method

The method is based on the equation $a - b = (a + 10) - (b + 10)$, with 10 added to both $a$ and $b$, which keeps the difference, $a - b$, the same. It is a harder method to explain to a child than the decomposition method, and Kennedy (1975) quite rightly pointed out that children have more difficulty remembering an algorithm they do not understand. It is also harder to provide multisensory experiences which clearly illustrate this algorithm. Despite these reservations, if the process can be mastered it is easy to reproduce. An 'easy' example may clarify the process, for example

$$320 - 90 \text{ becomes } (320 + 10) - (90 + 10) = 330 - 100.$$

The explanation could be developed from such examples.

Subtraction by equal additions is quicker, and probably easier, than decomposition as a mechanical process, but Kennedy's comment should be remembered as being particularly apposite for dyslexics, who often need a concrete base on which to build their understanding and memory.

## Mental arithmetic

The method of equal additions adjusts the numbers in the calculation and this is a strategy which can be extended into mental arithmetic. $342 - 197$ can be made an easier calculation by adding 3 to both numbers:

$$342 - 197 = 345 - 200.$$

This method is easier for some children than a similar procedure where the 197 is rounded up to 200, 200 is subtracted from 342 and 3 is added back onto the resultant 142.

A subtraction such as $411 - 115$ does require the latter strategy. The difference is approximately 300 but is less than 300. If 4 is added on to 411, then the subtraction gives an answer of 300. The added-on 4 now needs compensation, so $300 - 4 = 296$, the correct answer.

As before, the ability to perform mental arithmetic with facility is greatly enhanced by an understanding of the interrelationships between numbers and the relationship between addition and subtraction, so that $411 - 115$ is seen to be close to 300 and 197 is seen to be 3 short of 200. Such calculations also involve and develop estimation skills.

# Chapter 8
# Multiplication

## Introduction

This topic will be used to illustrate the use of a full programme of instruction. The principles of this structure are applicable to other topics. The work moves from a manipulative aid, which is a direct representation of the problem, to a model (in this case, area), to purely written symbols and an algorithm which links back to the concrete model. Whenever possible, more than one written method is given, so as to acknowledge the spectrum of cognitive styles. The multisensory introduction is used to lead into flexible cognitive processes and to give an introductory overview.

## The Special Case of Multiplying by 10 and Powers of 10

The first stage is to secure estimation skills. Estimation skills in multiplication (used, for example, to back up calculator work) centre on an ability to multiply by tens, hundreds, thousands, etc. In our experience this relatively basic operation needs frequent review (see Chapter 15 on the spiral construction of the Mark College mathematics programme).

The pattern of multiplying by 10 must be explained in terms of the basic concept and the implication on place value, rather than solely in terms of the purely mechanical action of 'adding on' zeros, a procedure which generates horror in the minds of mathematicians, yet is readily adopted by children (who tend to act so pragmatically).

The objective is to explain that multiplying by 10, 100, 1000 and so on moves numbers up in place value, but that the digits themselves do not change. To illustrate this, consider $536 \times 10$.

- $6 \times 10$. Use a place-value board and put six unit cubes in the units column. Remind the child of the 10-times table and the exchanging of ten blocks for unit cubes. Then ask the child to exchange each unit cube

84

for a ten block, placing the ten blocks in the tens column. Give the child a sheet of paper with place-value columns on it and ask him to write in numerals the 6 and the 60. Discuss the 60 being ten times bigger than the 6 and emphasise that the 6 has moved from the units column to the tens column (Figure 8.1a).

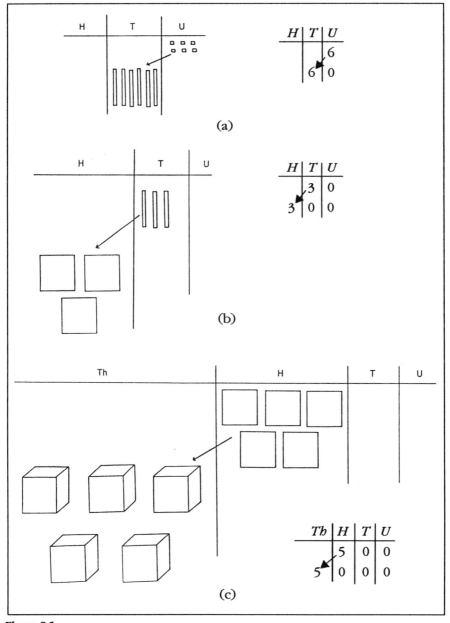

(a)

(b)

(c)

**Figure 8.1**

- $30 \times 10$. Repeat the process, but exchange three hundred blocks (squares) in the hundreds column for three ten blocks in the tens column (Figure 8.1b).

- $500 \times 10$. Repeat the process again exchanging five thousand blocks (cubes) for five hundred squares (Figure 8.1c).

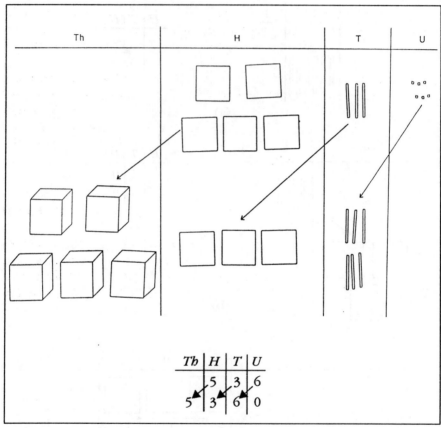

Figure 8.2

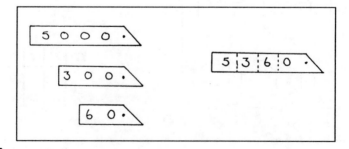

Figure 8.3

- 536 × 10. Repeat the process all in one example (Figure 8.2). Then discuss what has happened to each digit, the relevance numerically, the pattern, what has changed and what has not changed in the process. The procedure can be illustrated with place-value number arrows (Figure 8.3) as a further reinforcement of the concept.

It should now be possible for the child to explain equations such as $849 \times 10 = 8490$, including the significance of the zero in the units column, and to restate that the order of digits remains the same. As ever, this work includes a significant element of revisiting previous work and ideas.

A similar process can be used to teach $\times 100$ and $\times 1000$ and other powers of ten. Although not mathematically as sound as we would normally prefer, the relationship between the number of zeros in the multiplier and the number of extra zeros in the result should be pointed out. The child should also relate the number of place-value moves to the number of zeros in the multiplier.

The child should practise the work, using the base-ten blocks for some examples, place-value columns and (squared) paper for others. He should be encouraged to articulate his work and to review the underlying significance of the procedure.

It may be useful to extend multiplication by powers of ten to examples such as $\times 20$, $\times 60$, $\times 300$ and so on. The method advocated is a two-stage process, so that $\times 20$ is done as $\times 2$ then $\times 10$ (or $\times 10$ then $\times 2$). The child should compare the results of $\times 2$ with $\times 20$ by using base-ten blocks, e.g. $42 \times 20$:

$42 \times 10 = 420$ (Figure 8.4a)

$42 \times 2 = 84$ (Figure 8.4b)

giving

$42 \times 20 = 42 \times 2 \times 10 = 840$.

The child needs to realise that, if the multiplier is ten times bigger, then the result is ten times bigger. This procedure is, of course, similar to the times-table strategy for $\times 4$ of using $\times 2$ twice.

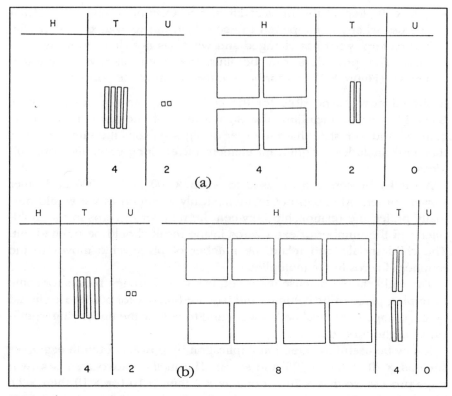

**Figure 8.4**

# Multiplication

Times-table facts are one digit times one digit operations. This chapter extends this to two digit times one digit and then to two digit times two digit and thus, by using the same models, to any multiplication. The model of multiplication used is area. This model is advocated because it can be extended into other aspects of multiplication (such as fraction times fraction) (Sharma, 1988).

### Introducing the model

The child needs some square counters (Figure 8.5). The three piles illustrate three lots of four. This can be discussed as repeated addition, $4 + 4 + 4$ leading to the more economical representation $3 \times 4$. The counters are then rearranged to represent area.

The concept of $a \times b$ as area can be discussed in real-life terms, such as carpet tiles, areas of wall for painting, etc.

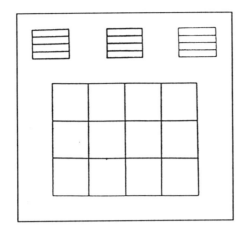

**Figure 8.5**

### Two digit times one digit

Consider $23 \times 4$. As with $\times 20$, the child is going to learn a two-stage procedure (not the same one). This procedure was used in the times-table chapter (Chapter 6) for the 2-times table, where, for example $7 \times 2$ was treated as $(5 \times 2) + (2 \times 2)$, a process of breaking down followed by building up again.

Set up the multiplication with base-ten blocks (Figure 8.6a). The area divides up into two sub-areas. One area is made up from tens blocks and the other area from unit blocks. The two areas can be physically separated to show $20 \times 4$ (Figure 8.6b) and $3 \times 4$ (Figure 8.6c). The two areas can then be brought back together to show $23 \times 4$ (Figure 8.6d).

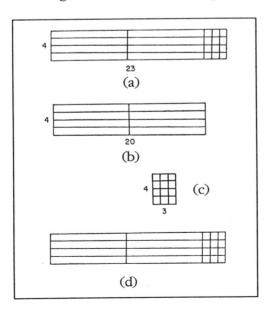

**Figure 8.6**

At each step the written symbols are shown to the child. The demonstration shows and separates the two partial products. The child should set up some areas for himself and show the partial products both as blocks and as written digits.

## Two digit times two digit

The model is again area. Consider the example $22 \times 31$. The inefficiency of repeated addition could be reviewed for this example:

$$22 + 22 + 22 + \ 22 + 22 + 22 + \ 22 + 22 + 22 + 22 + 22$$

$$+ \ 22 + 22 + 22 + 22 + 22 + 22 + 22 + 22 + 22 + 22$$

$$+ \ 22 + 22 + 22 + 22 + 22 + 22 + 22 + 22 + 22 + 22 \ .$$

Indeed, this overwhelming presentation would suggest some grouping and could be another route into the area model and the final algorithm.

1. Set up the multiplication in base-ten blocks (Figure 8.7a)). The blocks illustrate area. They are movable, so that the four sub-areas can be separated (Figure 8.7b). These partial products allow a difficult prob-

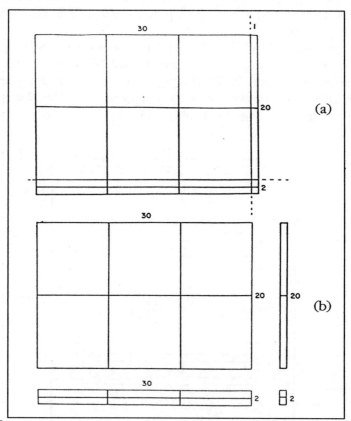

**Figure 8.7**

lem to be broken down into smaller, easier steps. The child can handle the blocks and physically break down the problem with the blocks, as well as with the written digits.

2. The four constituent areas are discussed, starting with the largest area, the area formed by the 'hundred squares'. This offers a first estimate. The blocks provide a very real model of this (Figure 8.8a). The estimation sum is written by the child in digits ($30 \times 20 = 600$).

3. The four areas are examined (Figure 8.8b). They are:

| $30 \times 20$ | tens $\times$ tens | $=$ | 600 |
| $1 \times 20$ | ones $\times$ tens | $=$ | 20 |
| $30 \times 2$ | tens $\times$ ones | $=$ | 60 |
| $1 \times 2$ | ones $\times$ ones | $=$ | 2 |
| | [total | $=$ | 682]. |

This algorithm is $(a + b)(c + d) = ac + ad + bc + bd$.

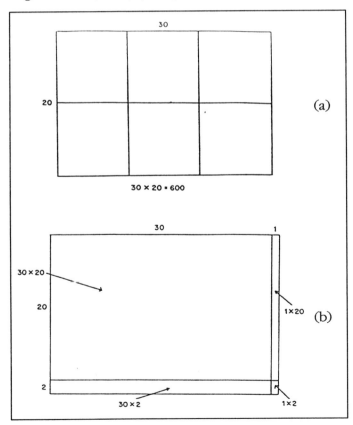

Figure 8.8

The child needs to see and handle each partial product in order to see that the area does break down into constituent parts. Each partial product should be written down in digits.

4. The problem is drawn to scale on squared paper by the child, and this will look like Figure 8.8b. The sub-divisions are drawn in, and the relationship between the areas and the numbers in the partial products is explained.

5. A problem is presented as numbers, e.g. $22 \times 31$. The partial products are written down and calculated. The child is asked to identify the 'estimate' partial product.

6. The problem is drawn to scale again on squared paper and only one sub-division is made, leaving two areas (Figure 8.9). In numbers the two areas are $20 \times 31$ and $2 \times 31$. The algorithm is based on $(a+b)c = ac+bc$.

The calculation becomes:

$$
\begin{array}{cc}
31 & \\
\times 22 & \\
\hline
620 & (31 \times 20) \\
62 & (31 \times 2) \\
\hline
682 & (31 \times 22)
\end{array}
$$

$$
\begin{array}{cc}
31 & 31 \\
\times 20 & \times 2 \\
\hline
620 & 62
\end{array}
$$

The child is still doing four multiplications as before, but he is combining two on each line of the calculation.

Compare the two methods as used for another example, $54 \times 23$:

$$
\begin{array}{ll}
54 & \\
\times 23 & \\
\hline
1000 & (50 \times 20) \\
80 & (4 \times 20) \\
150 & (50 \times 3) \\
12 & (4 \times 3) \\
\hline
1242 &
\end{array}
\qquad
\begin{array}{ll}
54 & \\
\times 23 & \\
\hline
1080 & (54 \times 20) \\
162 & (54 \times 3) \\
\hline
1242 &
\end{array}
$$

The child should chose the method which best helps his short-term memory, organisation and spatial problems.

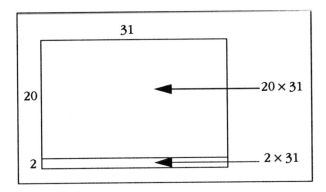

**Figure 8.9**

*Mnemonics may help the child*

1. FOIL (Figure 8.10)

   The First two digits are multiplied together: $50 \times 40$.

   The Outer two digits are multiplied together: $50 \times 3$.

   The Inner two digits are multiplied together: $2 \times 40$.

   The Last two digits are multiplied together: $2 \times 3$.

2. The smiley face (Figure 8.10). The lines join the numbers which have to be multiplied together. There can, however, be place-value problems with this mnemonic.

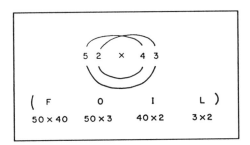

**Figure 8.10**

## Estimation

While calculators provide a relatively stress-free way of multiplying, dyslexics have a tendency to press the wrong number keys, get the numbers in the wrong order, use the wrong operation key or use the right operation key at the wrong time. A pre-estimate and a post-evaluation are, therefore, important.

The area model provides a good picture of how to estimate, based on the biggest sub-area plus or minus the other sub-areas. It also allows the child to evaluate his estimate and see if it is high, low or fairly accurate. Some examples will explain this.

- $33 \times 54$ (Figure 8.11a). This is estimated at $30 \times 50 = 1500$ and can be seen to be an underestimate, but reasonably close to the accurate answer.

- $42 \times 78$ (Figure 8.11b). Subtract to refine the estimate. Note that the 78 has been estimated *up* to 80 so that the length of the rectangle drawn is longer. The shaded part has to be subtracted if refined estimates are required. This, then, is estimated at $40 \times 80 = 3200$ and can be seen to be very close to the accurate answer with the extra $2 \times 40$ (which has to be subtracted) not quite compensating for the $2 \times 78$ (which has to be added).

- $51 \times 92$ (Figure 8.11c). Subtract to refine the estimate. Note that the 92 has been estimated *up* to 100. This is estimated at $50 \times 100 = 5000$ and can be seen to be an overestimate with $8 \times 50$ (which has to be subtracted) bigger than $1 \times 92$ (which has to be added).

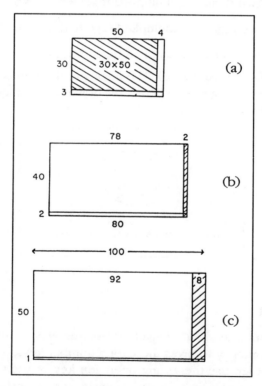

**Figure 8.11**

# Extension

The principle of the algorithm for a two digit times two digit calculation can be readily extended to three digit times three digit calculations and so on. The spatial organisation problems may require the child to work on squared paper (see Chapter 15), and in earlier examples the child may benefit from writing or articulating what each partial product means. Equally the principle of developing work from manipulative aids, through visual models, to symbol work is applicable to 'harder' examples.

These procedures integrate multisensory experiences with sound mathematical algorithms and provide the child with some concrete experiences and pictures which will help him to remember what might otherwise seem to him to be a meaningless random process. The structure provided by the identification of the partial products (and the number of partial products involved) helps the child and should help you, the teacher, with diagnosis of errors and subsequent remedial input.

# Chapter 9
# Division

## Introduction

In this chapter suggestions for teaching the concept of division and division by single-digit numbers and powers of ten are discussed. For more complex divisions, estimation followed by the use of a calculator is recommended, though an alternative algorithm to the traditional one is discussed, should you want to leave the child with at least one method for calculations.

The actual process of long division is very demanding on many of the skill areas that dyslexic students find most difficult. The algorithm traditionally used for long division requires good skills in sequencing, memory, knowledge of basic facts and spatial organisation.

It is worth considering the problems dyslexic pupils face in this particularly difficult topic. The extent of these difficulties may be alleviated by references to and building on other work the child has covered and by interrelating concepts (such as subtraction and division) so as to try and make old and new work mutually supportive. Once again, the child's existing knowledge makes a good baseline. You need to capitalise on existing knowledge and thus should begin with informal diagnostic work, which is intended to find out what the child knows and which examples and illustrations he relates to.

The language of division can lead to early problems and can be an initial block to understanding of the concept and processes of division. A typical early question could be, ' Divide 36 by 6' or ' 36 ÷ 6'. The order in which the numbers are stated is the opposite to the demands of the algorithm, $6\overline{)36}$.

Furthermore, 'divide' is an abstract word and children are more likely to be familiar with phrases such as 'How many 6's in 36?' or 'Share 36 between 6 people'. These phrases relate more readily to the manipulative materials and are easier for the child to grasp, so the move from concrete to symbolic requires the teacher to be aware of these language needs of the child, as well as of any lag in his conceptual development.

The spatial and organisational demands of division algorithms are considerable. The traditional algorithm for $6\overline{)378}$ requires the child to work from left to right, writing the answer at the top, working from the hundreds to the tens and then to the units and carrying down numbers as the problem proceeds. These requirements are almost directly opposite to those for addition, subtraction and multiplication. Furthermore, to help meet these directional demands, the child may well need support in getting the correct place values on the answer line. Extra support for this accuracy can be provided by teaching estimating skills and by encouraging the child to overview the question (which may include rephrasing it.)

## Introduction to Division

The initial aims are to introduce (or review) division in at least four ways: as sharing out or dividing up into parts; as finding out how many numbers in; as the converse of multiplication; and as repeated subtraction. An introductory activity of taking (small) numbers of counters and dividing them up into groups helps the child to see the processes of division in action and the interrelationship between division and subtraction. You can then extend the child's perception of the activity by structured questions and representation of the 'dividing up' actions.

*Example*

Take 12 counters and place them randomly on a table (Figure 9.1). Ask the child to count them. (Some children will group the counters automatically when they do this.) Then ask the child to share/divide them into in three groups.

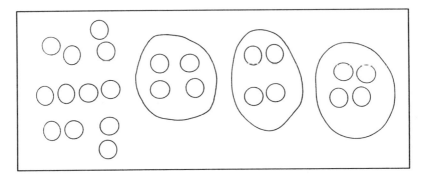

**Figure 9.1**

Ask the child to reorganise the groups into rows and columns. Then the following relationships can be examined as manipulatives and as equations:

Four lots of 3. (How many 3's in 12?)

Three lots of 4. (How many 4's in 12?)

3 goes into 12 four times.

12 divided by 3 gives 4.

Repeated subtraction of 3 from 12.

This work can be related back to the table square, so that its use as a division square can be taught. Repeated subtraction relates division to subtraction and acts as a first exposure to a later algorithm:

$$4 \times \square = 12 \qquad\qquad 12 \div 3 = 4$$

$$3 \times \square = 12$$

$$\frac{12}{3} = 4 \qquad\qquad 3 \overline{)12}^{\,4}$$

$$12 - 3 = 9$$

$$9 - 3 = 6$$

$$6 - 3 = 3$$

$$3 - 3 = 0.$$

Thus the child is seeing the relationship between division and multiplication, the idea of dividing up, the phrasing 'How many $x$ in $y$?', the concept of division as repeated subtraction and the idea of sharing equally. Simple division facts can be presented as multiplication facts with 'gaps' and the child can be shown how to use a table square to obtain division facts. Again the child is taught to use the interrelationships between numbers and operations in a way that makes maximum use of known facts, rather than the rote learning of seemingly unrelated facts.

Obviously many other examples besides 12 should be used, with the possibility of phasing out the (multisensory) manipulative aids as the child becomes more confident in his knowledge and understanding.

The relationship between the size/value of the divided number, divisor and answer can be shown by examples such as dividing 12 by a series of divisors: 12, 6, 4, 3, 2, 1. Work of this type (using, as ever, written presentation alongside manipulative work) leads the child towards estimation skills. At the least, the child is learning that the bigger the divisor, the smaller the answer.

## Dividing two-digit numbers by one-digit numbers, with remainder

Although the work described so far could be used to introduce a child to the topic of division, it is best considered as an early stage of remediation. For these early confidence-building stages, remainders provide less confusion than decimal or fraction answers. Thus $14 + 4$ is presented with counters (Figure 9.2). It is apparent that the answer is 3 and that there are two counters left over or remaining. 'Remainder' seems to be a reasonable name for these counters.

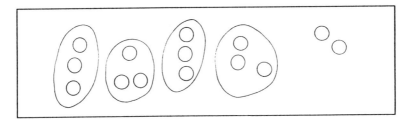

**Figure 9.2**

## Dividing two- and three-digit numbers with renaming (of tens and hundreds)

*Examples*

$65 + 5$

An efficient procedure for dividing 65 into five equal parts requires the child to progress from just counting out 65, unit by unit, into five groups. He has to learn how to start with 'How many 10's will be in each of the five parts?', then 'What do you do with the 10 left over and where do you bring in the 5 units from the 65'. In other words, this is quite a leap in skill and understanding. The demands of the algorithm on deficit areas are significant (see the Introduction to this chapter). Again the principle is to relate the symbols to a concrete base and make the algorithm relate to a manipulative procedure. A structured approach that pre-empts as many of the difficulties as possible and creates this concrete image for the child is advocated:

- 65 is presented in base-ten blocks (Figure 9.3a).

- Five tens are taken out, one to each of the five parts (Figure 9.3b).

- The 'left over' ten is traded for ten unit cubes and added to the existing five unit cubes.

- The 15 unit cubes are shared out, adding three unit cubes to each of the five parts making $10 + 3$, an answer of 13 (Figure 9.3d).

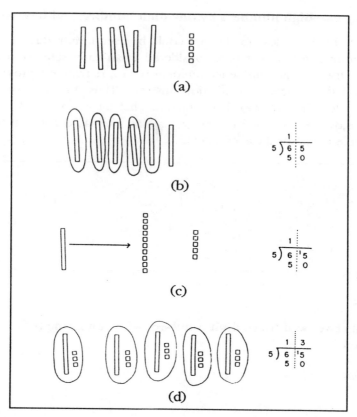

**Figure 9.3**

At each stage the written algorithm matches the base-ten manipulatives. You can explain the significance of each move and can relate it back to other work. For example, the need to trade tens for units is used in subtraction.

504 ÷ 4

- A similar structure is presented, with 504 shown in base-ten blocks. This time the first move is to take out four hundred blocks and place one in each part (Figure 9.4a).

- This leaves one hundred block, which is traded for 10 ten blocks, which are placed in the tens column. This highlights the previously empty tens column and emphasises the need to mark its presence in the answer line. Eight ten blocks are removed, two for each part (Figure 9.4b).

- The two remaining ten blocks are traded for unit cubes, giving 24 unit cubes to share into the four parts, six in each (Figure 9.4c).

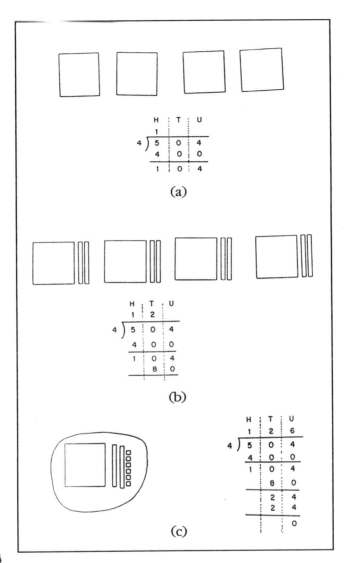

**Figure 9.4**

- The final answer is 126.

Note the use of place-value columns in the written version (given along-side the blocks in the parts of Figure 9.4). (Other suitable manipulative aids are money and bundles of cocktail sticks.)

Other examples should be used to consolidate this method. When the manipulative-aid stage is phased out, the use of the place-value lines should remain as it tends to eliminate the common errors of starting the answer in the wrong place or missing out a place as in $2\overline{)408}$ (often erron-eously answered as 24).

## Some alternative algorithms

Ashlock et al. (1983) offer two interesting alternatives, both based on repeated subtraction. Both require careful presentation. One is quite demanding on directional skills, but both offer a method which helps the child who cannot work out where to start. Both methods are based on subtracting multiples of the divisor. The pyramid algorithm (Figure 9.5a) allows the child to choose any estimate for his multiples. It also acts as a half-way house to the traditional algorithm, if that is the goal. The other algorithm leads to the answer mainly by multiplying the divisor by powers of ten (Figure 9.5b).

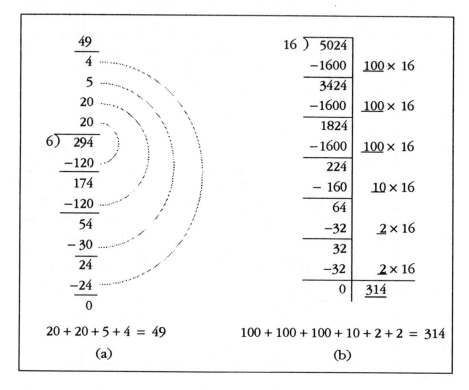

$$20 + 20 + 5 + 4 = 49$$

(a)

$$100 + 100 + 100 + 10 + 2 + 2 = 314$$

(b)

**Figure 9.5**

# Estimating

The ability to multiply the divisor by powers of ten can be used again to act as a useful estimating aid.

*Example*

3285 ÷ 5

The divisor is multiplied by increasing powers of ten and the product is compared with 3285:

$5 \times 10 = 50$

$5 \times 100 = 500$

$5 \times 1000 = 5000.$

So the answer will lie between 100 and 1000. It is, therefore, a three-digit answer and by comparing/evaluating 3285 with 500 and 5000 it can be seen that the quotient will be closer to 1000 than to 100. Again the link between division and multiplication is made and there is another chance for the child to reinforce his ability to multiply by powers of ten.

# Dividing by Powers of Ten

This is the converse of estimating. It requires an understanding of place value, so a review of this concept can be a precursor to the topic. The child needs to remember that the place a digit holds in a number controls its value by a power of ten (for example, in 58725, the 7 is the third number in, it is in the hundreds column and its value is $7 \times 100$ or 700).

Division by powers of ten produces a pattern which can be illustrated by activities where the pupil uses base-ten blocks to divide numbers into ten parts and thus is drawn to the conclusion that (as with multiplying by powers of ten) the numbers do not change, only their place value. At this early stage it is advisable to avoid answers which are decimals. A series of base-ten block activities leads to series such as:

| | | |
|---|---|---|
| $400 ÷ 10 = 40$ | $400 ÷ 100 = 4$ | $4000 ÷ 1000 = 4$ |
| $440 ÷ 10 = 44$ | $4000 ÷ 100 = 40$ | |
| $4000 ÷ 10 = 400$ | $4400 ÷ 100 = 44$ | |
| $4400 ÷ 10 = 440$ | | |
| $4440 ÷ 10 = 444$ | | |

It will almost certainly be necessary to use place-value columns to emphasise the way the numbers move. A structured programme of manipulative aids (base-ten blocks and/or money) and written digits should establish the idea of movement and values in the child's mind and lead him to some mnemonics. If this is so, then the move on to quotients that are decimals does not present such a difficult hurdle (see Chapter 12).

## Division by Multiples of Powers of Ten

Examples such as $4000 \div 20$, $3000 \div 2000$, $4500 \div 50$, etc. can solved by teaching the child to take a two-stage approach: dividing first by 10 and then by 2; by 1000 then by 3; by 10 then by 5. This can be a multisensory activity with base-ten blocks. (It also relates to the making of fractions such as 1/6 by a two-stage process: $\div 2$ and $\div 3$.)

## Conclusion

Further work should probably use calculators, providing that, as ever, there is an ability to estimate and check the answers. The work outlined in this chapter provides the child with the basic concept and the skills of division and the ability to estimate.

# Chapter 10
# Fractions, Decimals and Percentages: An Introduction

## Introduction

If mathematics is generally concerned with using numbers to describe things, then this chapter is about describing *parts* of things with numbers. There are important differences among the three alternative forms, otherwise fractions, decimals and percentages would not have evolved. Each of the three forms is described separately, its independent characteristics being covered in detail. The first aim is to help you establish, with the child, a good understanding of each form, and to avoid the possible misconceptions, many of which are specifically covered.

Of course, there are many similarities and equivalences between fractions, decimals and percentages – some text-books still refer to 'vulgar fractions' and 'decimal fractions'. Methods are covered for converting each form into each of the others, and in these the key values, such as $\frac{1}{2} = 0.5 = 50\%$, will be highlighted.

## Fractions

Fractions are the most basic way of describing parts of things. Thus, they are and have been taught in primary schools and there is an expectation from parents and perhaps some teachers that children should find fractions easy. Memories are being selective here, since fractions always were exceptionally difficult in their written form.

Many teachers and children use folding paper to establish how fractions work. It makes them easy to understand. In this book, this idea is taken further. The easy, folded-paper methods are allowed to dictate how fraction questions and answers should be written down. The written versions should then be just as easy to understand. Drawings of folded fractions provide a means of recording and communicating a point understood from the paper version. They form a step between the folded-paper fractions and the written fractions.

We recommend that roughly square shapes are folded and drawn at all times. The practice of using thin strips of paper masks the relationship, which it is invaluable to exploit, between forming fractions and multiplication of fractions (interpreted as two-dimensional in Chapter 11). That other popular alternative, the use of circles (or circular cakes), requires the understanding of harder concepts, such as angles and circle terms; also, how, for example, can a circular piece of paper be folded easily into equal fifths?

### Terminology

A fraction like $\dfrac{4}{5}$ will be referred to as 'part' of a whole thing. The fraction is made up of equal fifths, which will be referred to as 'segments', rather than parts of the fraction. This avoids the duplicate use of the word 'parts', and children will be familiar with the notion of segments of an orange.

The terms 'denominator' and 'numerator' should not be used with children, and will only be used in this book where they avoid clumsy circumlocutions.

### What is a fraction?

*Part of a whole thing*

- The piece of paper in Figure 10.1a has one fifth shaded in. It is divided into five equal segments and one is shaded, so the fraction is written as $\dfrac{1}{5}$.

- The fraction in Figure 10.1b shows three quarters. The written version is $\dfrac{3}{4}$.

Children can be asked to give the written form for other fractions, such as those shown in Figure 10.1c.

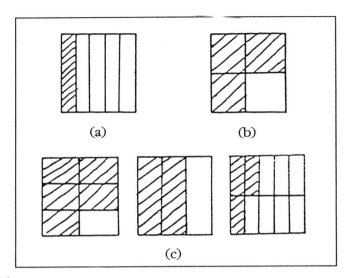

**Figure 10.1**

*Whole things divided into equal segments*

- Figure 10.2a shows a whole square of paper is five fifths (that's why they are called fifths). This is written as $\frac{5}{5}$ = 1 whole square.

  The number on the bottom of the fraction indicates both the number of segments and the size of the segments.

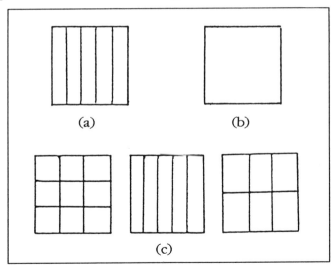

**Figure 10.2**

- The square in Figure 10.2b has been left whole. It can be written as $\frac{1}{1} = 1$ and called 1 whole.

  Children can be asked to write down the fraction for given examples, such as those shown in Figure 10.2c.

- The special name for the segments in Figure 10.3a – halves – should be highlighted.

- The segments in Figure 10.3b are usually known as quarters, but calling them fourths at the beginning tells children more about them.

- The version of fourths/quarters shown in Figure 10.3c should also be recognised.

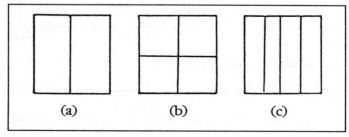

(a)            (b)            (c)

**Figure 10.3**

*More than one whole thing*

- Figure 10.4a shows two squares left whole. This can be written as $\frac{2}{1}$.

- Figure 10.4b shows two whole squares divided into quarters. This can be written as $2 \times \frac{4}{4} = \frac{8}{4}$.

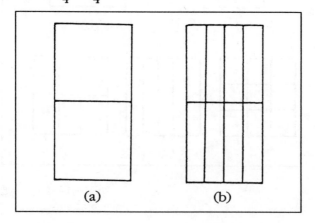

(a)                      (b)

**Figure 10.4**

## Making fractions

It is of the greatest importance that children make fractions themselves, by folding paper squares. This will help in the avoidance of such fundamental misconceptions as the idea that halving, halving and halving again will produce sixths. Demonstrably, it produces eighths. It will also help at future points of difficulty, if children can recall how the fractions were made.

*Halving procedure*

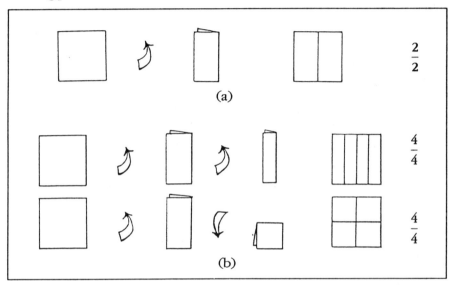

**Figure 10.5**

Figure 10.5a shows the folding procedure which produces halves. If the procedure is repeated, halving and halving again makes quarters (Figure 10.5b). Repeated halving produces a family of fractions, whose subsequent members are eighths, sixteenths, etc.

Other fractions require different folding procedures.

*Thirding procedure*

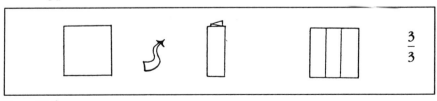

**Figure 10.6a**

The procedure shown in Figure 10.6a produces thirds. Repeating the procedure will produce a family of fractions, the next member of which is ninths.

*Fifthing procedure*

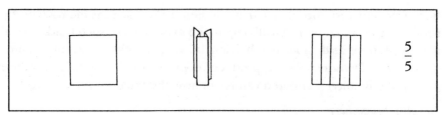

**Figure 10.6b**

The procedure shown in Figure 10.6b produces fifths and repeats to produce twentyfifths, etc.

*Other procedures*

A new procedure is required every time the number of segments is prime: $\dfrac{2}{2}, \dfrac{3}{3}, \dfrac{5}{5}, \dfrac{7}{7}$, etc.

In practice, halves, thirds and fifths are sufficient, because sevenths, elevenths, etc. are very rarely needed – and never desirable at the learning stage.

Some teachers refer to these folding procedures as 'machines', a term which can be legitimised through reference to automatic letter-folding machines.

## Other fractions

Other important fractions must be made using a combination of folding procedures.

• Sixths – made by halving and thirding in either order.

• Tenths – made by halving and fifthing in either order.

• Twelfths – made by halving, halving and thirding in any order.

• Twentieths – made by halving, halving and fifthing in any order.

Table 10.1 summarises how to make all the fractions it is worthwhile considering at this stage.

**Table 10.1**

| Fractions | Procedures | | | | | | |
|---|---|---|---|---|---|---|---|
| | Half | Half | Half | Half | Third | Third | Fifth |
| Halves | * | | | | | | |
| Thirds | | | | | * | | |
| Fourths/quarters | * | * | | | | | |
| Fifths | | | | | | | * |
| Sixths | * | | | | * | | |
| Eighths | * | * | * | | | | |
| Ninths | | | | | * | * | |
| Tenths | * | | | | | | * |
| Twelfths | * | * | | | * | | |
| Sixteenths | * | * | * | * | | | |
| Twentieths | * | * | | | | | * |

## Equal or equivalent fractions

Fractions are equal (or equivalent) if they cover the same amount/area of a paper square. For example, Figure 10.7 shows that $\frac{3}{4} = \frac{6}{8}$. The extra

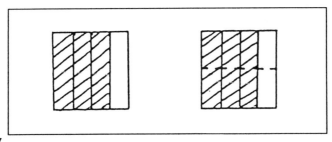

**Figure 10.7**

(horizontal) fold has produced twice as many segments and twice as many are shaded. The written format which gives the same effect is

$$\frac{3}{4} = \frac{3 \times 2}{4 \times 2} = \frac{6}{8}.$$

Formally, it is permissible to multiply the top and bottom by the same number. There are many different forms of exercise for establishing this concept.

1. Give the written form for the two equal fractions shown in Figure 10.8a.

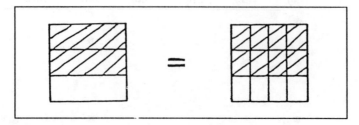

**Figure 10.8a**

2. Draw in the extra fold lines in Figure 10.8b to show that $\dfrac{1}{2} = \dfrac{3}{6}$.

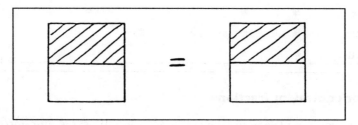

**Figure 10.8b**

3. Write the correct numbers in the empty boxes:

$$\frac{1}{3} = \frac{1 \times 5}{3 \times 5} = \frac{\square}{\square} \ ;$$

$$\frac{3}{5} = \frac{3 \times \square}{5 \times 2} = \frac{6}{\square} \ ;$$

$$\frac{3}{8} = \frac{3 \times \square}{8 \times \square} = \frac{9}{\square} \ ;$$

$$\frac{3}{4} = \frac{3 \times \square}{4 \times \square} = \frac{\square}{16} \ .$$

## Simplifying fractions

*Example*

In the example shown in Figure 10.9, it is possible to divide all the tenths into groups of two, as shown. The shaded four are divided into groups of two at the same time. The written format which gives this effect is:

$$\frac{4}{10} = \frac{4 \div 2}{10 \div 2} = \frac{2}{5}.$$

Formally, it is permissible to divide the top and the bottom by the same number.

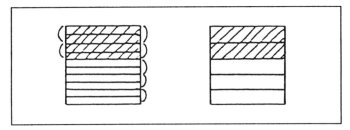

**Figure 10.9**

A practical problem, here, is to decide what number to use for dividing the top and the bottom, i.e. into what size groups can the segments be divided. Prime factors can be used, or trial and error (based on a knowledge of the multiplication/division facts), but the method consistent with the philosophy of this book is to try the numbers used in forming the original segments by folding.

In the example above, tenths would have been formed by folding into halves and fifths. Therefore, dividing into groups of two or five should be tried. Of these, only the groups of two work for the shaded segments, and so the fraction is in its 'lowest terms', when this has been done.

*Example*

Simplify $\frac{8}{12}$. For this example, the twelfths would be formed by folding into halves, halves and thirds. Therefore, dividing by 2, 2 and 3 should be attempted:

$$\frac{8}{12} = \frac{8 \div 2}{12 \div 2} = \frac{4}{6}$$

$$= \frac{4 \div 2}{6 \div 2} = \frac{2}{3}.$$

Dividing top and bottom by 3 does not work, so the fraction is as simple as it can be made.

Since halving and halving again produces quarters, a short cut would be to try dividing directly into groups of four, as illustrated in Figure 10.10.

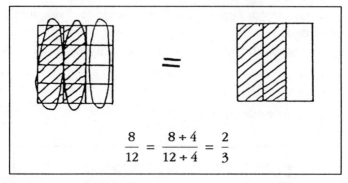

$$\frac{8}{12} = \frac{8+4}{12+4} = \frac{2}{3}$$

**Figure 10.10**

There are many different forms of exercise for establishing this concept.

1. What are the folding steps which would make the following fraction in Figure 10.11?

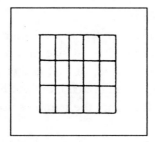

**Figure 10.11**

2. Write the correct numbers in the empty boxes:

$$\frac{5}{10} = \frac{5+5}{10+5} = \frac{\square}{\square} \; ;$$

$$\frac{4}{12} = \frac{4+4}{12+\square} = \frac{1}{\square} \; ;$$

$$\frac{2}{6} = \frac{2+\square}{6+\square} = \frac{1}{\square} \; ;$$

$$\frac{8}{20} = \frac{8+\square}{20+\square} = \frac{4}{\square} = \frac{4+\square}{\square+\square} = \frac{\square}{5} \; ;$$

$$\frac{6}{10} = \frac{6+\square}{10+\square} = \frac{\square}{\square} \; .$$

# Decimals

Decimals are parts of a whole thing.

Where a number also contains some whole things, the decimal part is separated by a decimal point, e.g. 37.651

There is a sense in which decimals are just specific fractions – the first column after the decimal point representing tenths, the second representing hundredths, etc. However, because of this, each column is ten times the previous column, and so decimals are a continuation of the whole number system. They demonstrate this property when a number is carried in an addition, for example, or when a decimal is multiplied by 10.

### First place as tenths

This can be demonstrated well with a measuring exercise. Consider the following length *AB* marked against a scale (Figure 10.12).

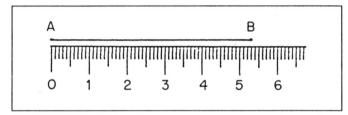

**Figure 10.12**

- Each large unit on the scale (cm) is divided into 10 smaller units (mm).

- Each smaller unit will be $\dfrac{1}{10}$ of a large unit

- The length *AB* is 53 small units and $5\dfrac{3}{10}$ large units

- If *AB* is written as 5.3 large units, then .3 means $\dfrac{3}{10}$ and the first number after the decimal point represents tenths.

This convention can be established and reinforced for children by having them measure a series of modest lengths and write their answers in centimetres as both fractions and decimals. If centimetres and millimetres are too small, a ruler graduated in inches and tenths of an inch will give a useful increase in size.

### Second place as hundredths

This can be demonstrated with a money example.

$$100\text{p} = £1$$

$$10\text{p} = £\frac{1}{10}$$

$$1\text{p} = £\frac{1}{100}.$$

Almost all children will accept and understand the above equivalents for money units. The amount of money illustrated in Figure 10.13 is written in pence at the top and pounds at the bottom.

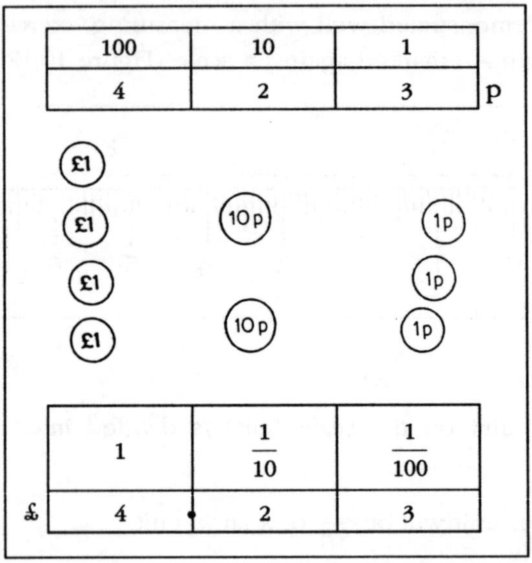
100 10 1
4 2 3 p
£1
£1
10p
1p
1p
£1
10p
1p
£1
1 1/10 1/100
£ 4 • 2 3

**Figure 10.13**

With the amount of money in pounds, the decimal point takes up its familiar position. Figure 10.13 confirms that the first column after the decimal point represents tenths and shows that the second column represents hundredths.

A good exercise for establishing and reinforcing this convention is to ask children to convert various quantities of pennies into pounds, written as both decimals and fractions, e.g.

$$587\text{p} = £5.87 = £5\frac{87}{100}.$$

Fractions which simplify should be avoided at this stage, because, after simplification, they would produce something other than hundredths.

### Further decimal places

Once the fraction equivalents are established for the first and second places of decimals, it is relatively easy for children to accept the next place as thousandths, and so on. A reminder that the familiar whole number column headings are Ones, Tens, Hundreds, Thousands, etc. is usually helpful.

It is worthwhile emphasising here that decimal place-value difficulties (like difficulties with whole number place values) are dramatically reduced if children can be persuaded to write their examples down in columns with headings.

### Converting decimals to fractions

As was outlined earlier, decimals are composed of the specific fractions $\frac{1}{10}$, $\frac{1}{100}$, $\frac{1}{1000}$, etc., depending on the column(s) in which they are written. To convert them back to fractions, it is necessary simply to read off which of these columns they reach. Examples are given in Figure 10.14.

| $\frac{1}{10}$ | $\frac{1}{100}$ | $\frac{1}{1000}$ | |
|---|---|---|---|
| 3 | | | $\frac{3}{10}$ |
| 3 | 7 | | $\frac{37}{100}$ |
| 0 | 9 | | $\frac{9}{100}$ |
| 7 | 8 | 9 | $\frac{789}{1000}$ |
| 0 | 0 | 7 | $\frac{7}{1000}$ |
| 0 | 2 | 3 | $\frac{23}{1000}$ |

**Figure 10.14**

For those children who, during this last example, question why the 2 (in the second column) is not seen as $\dfrac{2}{100}$, there follows an explanation (which slightly anticipates addition of fractions).

$$.023 = \begin{array}{c} \dfrac{2}{100} \\[4pt] + \\[4pt] \dfrac{3}{1000} \end{array} = \begin{array}{c} \dfrac{20}{1000} \\[4pt] + \\[4pt] \dfrac{3}{1000} \end{array} = \dfrac{23}{1000}$$

### Examples which can be simplified

After some decimals have been converted into fractions, they can be simplified.

$$= \frac{8}{10} = \frac{8 \div 2}{10 \div 2} = \frac{4}{5}$$

$$= \frac{45}{100} = \frac{45 \div 5}{100 \div 5} = \frac{9}{20}$$

$$= \frac{4}{1000} = \frac{4 \div 4}{1000 \div 4} = \frac{1}{250}$$

### Use of the number 25

In many cases, where decimals have been converted into fractions, and are to be simplified, the ability to divide (top and bottom) by 25 is very useful, as a short cut. There are two in 50, three in 75, four in every 100 and so 40 in every 1000, e.g.

$$.375 = \frac{375}{1000} = \frac{375 \div 25}{1000 \div 25} = \frac{15}{40} = \frac{15 \div 5}{40 \div 5} = \frac{3}{8}$$

### Special decimals

A few decimals convert and simplify to very important fractions. It is desirable for these to be remembered by heart:

$$.1 = \frac{1}{10} \qquad .01 = \frac{1}{100} \qquad .001 = \frac{1}{1000}$$

$$.5 = \frac{1}{2} \qquad .25 = \frac{1}{4} \qquad .75 = \frac{3}{4} \qquad .2 = \frac{1}{5}.$$

## The significance of zeros

Zeros in certain positions are very important, whereas others are unimportant or optional. As with whole numbers, it is the zeros that hold other numbers in their right places which have significance. The following pairs of examples can be used to demonstrate the possibilities:

| $\frac{1}{10}$ | $\frac{1}{100}$ | |
|---|---|---|
| 7 | | $= \frac{7}{10}$ |
| 0 | 7 | $= \frac{7}{100}$ |

The zero in .07 gives it a different value from .7.

| $\frac{1}{10}$ | $\frac{1}{100}$ | $\frac{1}{1000}$ | |
|---|---|---|---|
| 1 | 0 | 9 | $= \frac{109}{1000}$ |
| 1 | 9 | | $= \frac{19}{100}$ |

The zero in .109 again affects its value, because it pushes the 9 into a different place.

| $\frac{1}{10}$ | $\frac{1}{100}$ | |
|---|---|---|
| 3 | | $= \frac{3}{10}$ |
| 3 | 0 | $= \frac{30}{100} = \frac{3}{10}$ |

The zero in .30 makes no ultimate difference to its value, although there are ways in which it can sometimes be made useful, as will be shown later.

When a decimal, such as .92 has no whole number part, it is usually written in the form 0.92, with an optional zero at the front, as a matter of style. As long as children are having difficulty with decimals, simplicity is more important than style, so this should be avoided. In this chapter, such zeros have been omitted, for this reason.

In general, just as for whole numbers, the significant zeros are located between other numbers, or between a number and the decimal point. The unimportant or optional zeros are to be found beyond those numbers furthest from the decimal point.

## Comparing decimals

'Which decimal is bigger .87 or .135?' In answer to this question, many children will answer .135, because they see 135 as bigger than 87. Of course, they are not comparing like with like, because the 135 are thousandths whereas the 87 are hundredths. By way of explanation, all that is necessary is to write the decimals in their columns and make them the same 'length' by using optional zeros:

| $\dfrac{1}{10}$ | $\dfrac{1}{100}$ | $\dfrac{1}{1000}$ |
|---|---|---|
| 8 | 7 | 0 |
| 1 | 3 | 5 |

This process has the same effect as making segment sizes the same for fractions. Now the 870 is clearly bigger than the 135.

Some children have a similar problem understanding why .25 is halfway between .2 and .3, both of which may seem smaller. The column headings and optional zeros can help again:

| $\dfrac{1}{10}$ | $\dfrac{1}{100}$ |
|---|---|
| 2 | 0 |
| 2 | 5 |
| 3 | 0 |

Quite clearly, 25 hundredths is half-way between 20 hundredths and 30 hundredths.

Another approach to these and other similar problems is to explain with a decimal number line, such as is shown in Figure 10.15. This number line shows quite clearly that .87 is bigger than .135. The equivalent fractions above the line provide further justification. It also shows that .25 lies half-way between .2 and .3, another such situation being observable at .865, which is half-way between .86 and .87.

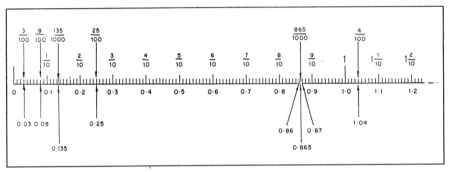

**Figure 10.15** Number line for decimals

### Decimal number sequences

Decimal number sequences can be regarded as extended extracts from a number line, such as that above. If the extracts are selected carefully, they can provide a very convincing alternative way of looking at problem areas that have not been fully understood. One such problem area is tackled below. Consider the following sequence:

> 2.97, 2.98, 2.99,     .

Those children who have not properly taken on board the message that decimals behave in their columns, just like ordinary whole numbers, may make the mistake of supposing that the next decimal in the sequence is 2.100. They have not understood that the 1 from the 100 will be carried across the decimal point to produce 3.00. One way to clarify the situation is to suggest that the decimal point could be temporarily ignored, where-upon the 299 would naturally be followed by 300. Perhaps a more satis-factory method, and certainly a more interesting method for the children, is to challenge them with a decimal number sequence where the missing number is in the middle of the sequence. The above sequence might become:

> 2.97, 2.98, 2.99,     , 3.01, 3.02, 3.03

The opportunity now exists to find the missing decimal more easily, by approaching it from the other direction. Working towards it downwards gives 3.03, 3.02, 3.01, and then quite naturally 3.00. Furthermore, all kinds of very sound ideas about checking answers by working backwards and the reciprocity of addition and subtraction are being quietly covered.

Each of the following sequences straddles a different awkward region, where the numbers in parentheses would be left out for the children to find:

> 1.7, 1.8, 1.9, (2.0), (2.1), 2.2, 2.3
>
> 7.3, 7.2, (7.1), (7.0), 6.9, 6.8
>
> 8.8, 8.6, 8.4, 8.2, (8.0), 7.8, 7.6, 7.4
>
> 39.7, 39.8, 39.9, (40.0), (40.1), 40.2, 40.3
>
> 20.03, 20.02, (20.01), (20.00), (19.99), 19.98, 19.97.

## Converting fractions to decimals

Some fractions are very simple to convert into decimals, because they are already tenths, hundredths or thousandths. They slot into the decimal columns immediately, like the examples below:

|   |   | $\frac{1}{10}$ | $\frac{1}{100}$ | $\frac{1}{1000}$ |
|---|---|---|---|---|
| $\frac{1}{10}$ = | • | 1 |   |   |
| $\frac{23}{100}$ = | • | 2 | 3 |   |
| $\frac{7}{100}$ = | • | 0 | 7 |   |
| $\frac{3}{1000}$ = | • | 0 | 0 | 3 |
| $\frac{29}{1000}$ = | • | 0 | 2 | 9 |
| $\frac{527}{1000}$ = | • | 5 | 2 | 7 |

There are other fractions, which can easily be made into tenths, hundredths or thousandths, as shown with the following examples:

| | | $\dfrac{1}{10}$ | $\dfrac{1}{100}$ | $\dfrac{1}{1000}$ |
|---|---|---|---|---|
| $\dfrac{2}{5} = \dfrac{2 \times 2}{5 \times 2} = \dfrac{4}{10} =$ | | 4 | | |
| $\dfrac{3}{4} = \dfrac{3 \times 25}{4 \times 25} = \dfrac{75}{100} =$ | | 7 | 5 | |
| $\dfrac{1}{20} = \dfrac{1 \times 5}{20 \times 5} = \dfrac{5}{100} =$ | | 0 | 5 | |
| $\dfrac{7}{8} = \dfrac{7 \times 125}{8 \times 125} = \dfrac{875}{1000} =$ | | 8 | 7 | 5 |

The final example, $\dfrac{7}{8}$ in the table above, depends for its conversion on the knowledge that $8 \times 125 = 1000$. The likely absence of this knowledge would push this conversion into the most difficult category, along with fractions like $\dfrac{5}{9}$. There is no way in which $\dfrac{5}{9}$ can be converted into tenths, hundredths or thousandths. For such an example, it is necessary to regard $\dfrac{5}{9}$ as $5 \div 9$, and to perform a decimal division, which is beyond the scope of this chapter, so such conversions are covered in Chapter 12.

## Percentages

Percentages are another way of describing parts of whole things.

'Per cent' means 'out of 100'. For example, 1 per cent means 1 out of a 100, which can also be written as 1/100. In essence, 'percentages are hundredths'. The sign for per cent, %, seems to be constructed from a 1, a 0 and another 0, so it behaves as a perpetual and valuable reminder of the importance of 100. Clearly, since percentages are hundredths, it is a simple matter to convert between percentages and fractions. Moreover, since hundredths constitute one of the decimal column headings, it is also relatively easy to convert between percentages and decimals.

### Percentages and whole things

Writing down whole things in terms of percentages is slightly more difficult than with fractions or decimals, where whole numbers are just written separately, in front. However, there is subsequently much less need to manipulate the percentages, so the difficulty carries no further.

A whole thing is $\frac{100}{100}$, which is 100%. Every whole thing is 100%, and so, for example, the whole number 5 is 500%.

# A Global Model for Percentages, Fractions and Decimals

Figure 10.16 shows a whole square divided into 100 equal segments. Each segment is $\frac{1}{100}$, or 1%, or .01 (1 in the hundredths column). These can be represented physically by the unit bricks in Dienes apparatus. Each column is $\frac{1}{10}$, or 10%, or .1 (1 in the tenths column). These can be represented by 'longs'. The whole square is 100%, or 1 whole number, and could be represented by a 'flat'.

Percentages are a rather more palatable way of expressing parts of whole things, for most people.

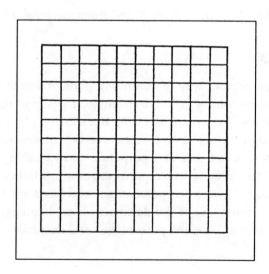

**Figure 10.16**

1. Because they are so small, any part of a whole thing will contain a workable number of them.

2. Understood to be hundredths, they are fractions written without a denominator, or decimals without the need for the decimal point.

3. More generally, it seems easier for most people to visualise 39%, for example, as 39 out of *their* picture of 100, rather than $\frac{39}{100}$ or .39.

4. Percentages are much easier to compare.

**Comparing percentages**

Unlike fractions, which can have segments of any size, or decimals, which can be tenths, hundredths, thousandths, etc., percentages all have the same segment size – they are all hundredths. Their numerical values can therefore be compared in a straightforward way – the bigger the number, the bigger the percentage (and the bigger the part that it represents).

*Examples*

- 38% is bigger than 26% (by 12%) (Figure 10.17).

- 19% is smaller than 82% (by 61%).

- 31% is bigger than 7.25%.

- 135% is bigger than 87%.

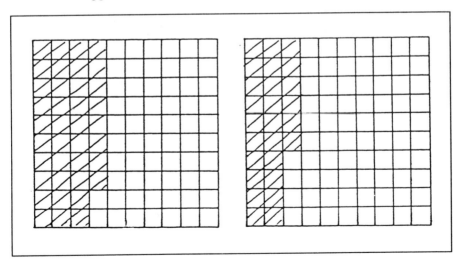

**Figure 10.17**

## Converting percentages to fractions

Percentages are 'understood' to be hundredths, so converting them to fractions is simply a matter of writing them with 100 on the bottom.

*Examples*

- $27\% = \dfrac{27}{100}$ (Figure 10.18).

- $127\% = 1\,\dfrac{27}{100}$.

- $91\% = \dfrac{91}{100}$.

- $9\% = \dfrac{9}{100}$.

Sometimes the fraction obtained can be simplified.

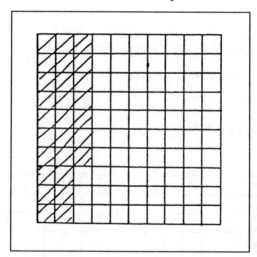

**Figure 10.18**

*Examples*

$$45\% \;=\; \frac{45}{100} \;=\; \frac{45+5}{100+5} \;=\; \frac{9}{20} \quad \text{(Figure 10.19)}.$$

$$62\% \;=\; \frac{62}{100} \;=\; \frac{62+2}{100+2} \;=\; \frac{31}{50}.$$

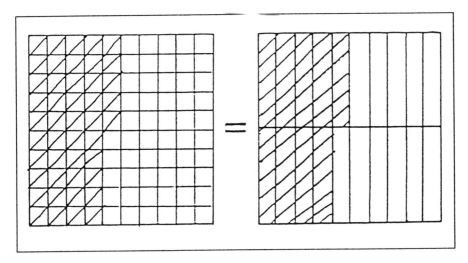

**Figure 10.19**

$$70\% \quad = \frac{70}{100} = \frac{70 \div 10}{100 \div 10} = \frac{7}{10}.$$

$$75\% \quad = \frac{75}{100} = \frac{75 \div 25}{100 \div 25} = \frac{3}{4}.$$

$$5\% \quad = \frac{5}{100} = \frac{5 \div 5}{100 \div 5} = \frac{1}{20}.$$

Some percentages produce fractions that take many steps to simplify. Such simplifications rarely occur elsewhere, and so they are covered here.

*Example*

$$12.5\% \quad = \frac{12.5}{100} = \frac{12.5 \times 10}{100 \times 10} = \frac{125}{1000}.$$

$$= \frac{125 \div 25}{1000 \div 25} = \frac{5}{40}.$$

$$= \frac{5 \div 5}{40 \div 5} = \frac{1}{8}.$$

(See Chapter 12 for multiplying decimals by 10.)

*Example*

$$33\,\tfrac{1}{3}\,\% \;=\; \frac{33\tfrac{1}{3}}{100} \;=\; \frac{33\tfrac{1}{3}\times 3}{100\times 3} \;=\; \frac{\dfrac{100}{3}\times 3}{300}.$$

$$=\; \frac{100}{300} \;=\; \frac{100\div 100}{300\div 100}.$$

$$=\; \frac{1}{3}.$$

(See Chapter 11 for multiplication of fractions.)

## Converting fractions to percentages

When fractions are hundredths, a % can replace the 100 in the denominator.

*Examples*

$$\frac{83}{100} \;=\; 83\%.$$

$$2\frac{83}{100} \;=\; 283\%.$$

$$\frac{7}{100} \;=\; 7\%.$$

Some fractions have first to be changed into hundredths. (A similar step was necessary in converting fractions to decimals.)

*Examples*

$$\frac{1}{2} \;=\; \frac{1\times 50}{2\times 50} \;=\; \frac{50}{100} \;=\; 50\%\,\text{(Figure 10.20)}.$$

$$\frac{2}{5} \;=\; \frac{2\times 20}{5\times 20} \;=\; \frac{40}{100} \;=\; 40\%.$$

$$\frac{12}{25} \;=\; \frac{12\times 4}{25\times 4} \;=\; \frac{48}{100} \;=\; 48\%.$$

$$\frac{37}{50} \;=\; \frac{37\times 2}{50\times 2} \;=\; \frac{74}{100} \;=\; 74\%.$$

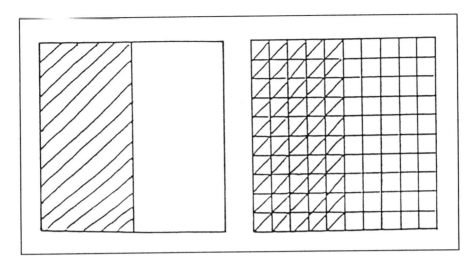

**Figure 10.20**

At times, children will be unable to change the fraction into hundredths, because they do not know the multiplier that will make the denominator 100. Finding this multiplier becomes the first step. Consider $\frac{17}{20}$:

$$\frac{17}{20} = \frac{17 \times ?}{20 \times ?} = \frac{?}{100}.$$

It is required to identify how many 20's in 100. Put this way, it becomes evident that 100 needs to be divided into 20's. Since $100 \div 20 = 5$, it is now possible to multiply top and bottom by 5 and obtain hundredths:

$$\frac{17}{20} = \frac{17 \times 5}{20 \times 5} = \frac{85}{100} = 85\%.$$

Sometimes there is no whole number that will multiply the denominator to produce 100. The required multiplier is a decimal. Proper consideration for decimals is given in Chapter 12, but an example is dealt with here, for completeness. Consider $\frac{5}{16}$. Now $100 \div 16 = 6.25$, and so this is the required multiplier:

$$\frac{5}{16} = \frac{5 \times 6.25}{16 \times 6.25} = \frac{31.25}{100} = 31.25\%.$$

$\dfrac{5}{16}$ is a very simple fraction, which has become the rather clumsy per-

centage 31.25%. Nevertheless, this form will give some people a much better understanding of the part of a whole thing represented.

### Converting percentages to decimals

Percentages are understood to be hundredths, and the second column of decimals is understood to be for hundredths. Therefore it is a simple matter to write a whole-number percentage in the decimal columns. It is required to finish in the hundredths column.

*Examples*

| | $\dfrac{1}{10}$ | $\dfrac{1}{100}$ | $\dfrac{1}{1000}$ | $\dfrac{1}{10000}$ |
|---|---|---|---|---|
| 28% = | 2 | 8 | | (Figure 10.21) |
| 72% = | 7 | 2 | | |
| 50% = | 5 | 0 | | |
| | 5 | | | |
| 8% = | 0 | 8 | | |
| 31.25% = | 3 | 1 | 2 | 5 |

The final example above shows the harder decimal percentage which was converted from $\dfrac{5}{16}$. Exceptionally, it does not finish in the hundredths column, because of the .25% on the end. This needs extra decimal places, reaching to the ten thousandths, because

$$.25\% = \frac{0.25}{100} = \frac{0.25 \times 100}{100 \times 100} = \frac{25}{10000}.$$

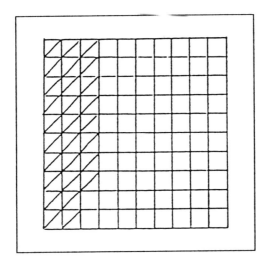

**Figure 10.21**

## Converting decimals to percentages

The second column of decimals is for hundredths. Therefore, any decimal, which can be 'lifted' entirely out of the first two columns of decimals, can be written immediately as a percentage.

*Examples*

|  | $\dfrac{1}{10}$ | $\dfrac{1}{100}$ | $\dfrac{1}{1000}$ |  |
|----|----|----|----|----|
|  | 2 | 5 |  | = 25% |
|  | 9 | 7 |  | = 97% |
|  | 0 | 5 |  | = 5% |
|  | 1 | 0 |  | = 10% |
| so | 1 | 8 |  | = 18% |

If the decimal contains more than two places, then the percentage will have to be extended to contain them.

*Examples*

| | 1 | $\frac{1}{10}$ | $\frac{1}{100}$ | $\frac{1}{1000}$ | $\frac{1}{10000}$ | |
|---|---|---|---|---|---|---|
| | | 6 | 6 | | | = 66% |
| so | | 6 | 6 | 6 | 6 | = 66.66% |
| | | 3 | 7 | | | = 37% |
| so | | 3 | 7 | 5 | | = 37.5% |
| | | 1 | 8 | | | = 18% |
| so | 4 | 1 | 8 | | | = 418% |

## Special percentages

The following list shows the equivalent percentages, fractions and decimals for the most important parts of a whole thing:

$$\frac{1}{2} = 50\% = .5$$

$$\frac{1}{4} = 25\% = .25$$

$$\frac{3}{4} = 75\% = .75$$

$$\frac{1}{10} = 10\% = .1$$

$$\frac{1}{5} = 20\% = .2$$

$$\frac{1}{3} = 33\frac{1}{3}\%$$

$$= 33.3\% = .333$$

$$\frac{2}{3} = 66^2/_3\%$$

$$= 66.6\% = .666$$

$$\frac{1}{100} = 1\% = .01$$

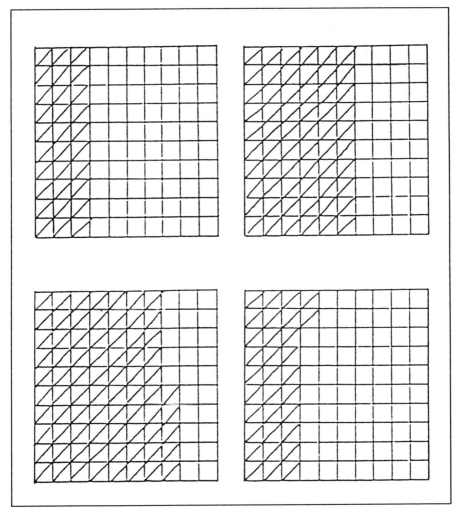

**Figure 10.22**

# A Global Exercise with Fractions, Percentages and Decimals

In order to practise the various conversion processes detailed in this chapter, the child should give the written forms of the shaded parts on diagrams, such as those shown in Figure 10.22. He should write percentages, decimals and fractions (simplified where possible).

# Chapter 11
# Operating with Fractions

## Introduction

Work with simple fractions epitomises the argument 'Mathematics is easy, only writing it down is hard'. For example, as we shall show, it is very easy to make $3\frac{1}{4} + 1\frac{1}{2}$ into $4\frac{3}{4}$ using the paper-folding model advocated in this book for introducing fractions, but the written version, which carries with it a complex and virtually unjustifiable algorithm, seems very difficult indeed by comparison. The work in this chapter is designed to link the 'doing' with the 'writing down' with the aim of making them equally easy. The paper-folding model also provides a visual and kinaesthetic image to help the child recall and use the algorithm correctly.

As in Chapter 10, the ideas illustrated and substantiated by paper folding show the child what the written-down version should be, so that the written version of the problem relates directly to the concrete model. Thus, at a point of difficulty with a written problem there will be a parallel paper-folding procedure to support memory (or conceptual difficulties).

Here, as elsewhere in this book, the structure brought by these models and the procedures are intended to contribute towards the pupil's overall understanding of the algorithms and concepts. The use of folded-paper fractions is often clear enough for the diagrams or examples to speak for themselves, and thus the minimum amount of explanatory text is needed. As in other chapters, you must use your experience of the child to blend the work to suit the individual. The basic structure is, however, best left intact.

## Making Segment Sizes the Same

It will become apparent at points in this chapter that if two or more fractions are to be compared, added or subtracted, their segments must be the same size. Generally, their segments will not be the same size, but there is a method of making them so, which is fully consistent with the philosophy of this book. It depends on the argument that for segments to be made the same size, the fractions must be made to undergo the same paper-folding steps. Each fraction must be given the folds it does not already share with the others. The folding can be real, drawn, imagined or written, but the objective will be a situation where all fractions have been through the same folding steps. The experience gained earlier, in actually making fractions, will be valuable here.

### Examples

- Consider the fractions $^7/_8$ and $^3/_4$ (Figure 11.1a).

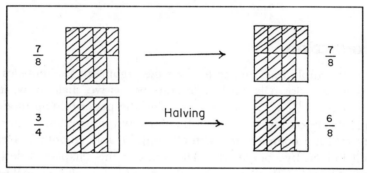

**Figure 11.1a**

| | Folding it has had | Folding it now needs |
|---|---|---|
| $^7/_8$ | Halving, halving, halving | – |
| $^3/_4$ | Halving, halving | Halving |

The written version is shown in Figure 11.1b. The folded-paper diagram and the written version are now showing eighths as the segment size for both fractions.

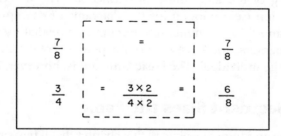

**Figure 11.1b**

- Consider the fractions $^3/_4$ and $^2/_3$ (Figure 11.2a). $^3/_4$ has been through halving and halving and $^2/_3$ has been through thirding. $^3/_4$ now needs thirding; $^2/_3$ now needs halving and halving. The

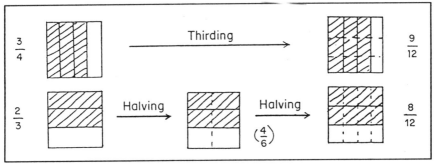

**Figure 11.2a**

written version which gives this effect is shown in Figure 11.2b. Now twelfths is the segment size for both fractions. Notice that it is unnecessary to know in advance that the shared segment size will be twelfths.

$$\frac{3}{4} \qquad = \qquad \frac{3 \times 3}{4 \times 3} \qquad = \qquad \frac{9}{12}$$

$$\frac{2}{3} \qquad = \frac{2 \times 2}{3 \times 2} \quad = \frac{4}{6} \quad = \frac{4 \times 2}{6 \times 2} \quad = \frac{8}{12}$$

**Figure 11.2b**

- Consider $\frac{5}{6}$ and $\frac{9}{10}$ . After considering how they were formed, it is evident that $\frac{5}{6}$ now needs fifthing and $\frac{9}{10}$ needs thirding. This time using the written form only gives

$$\frac{5}{6} = \frac{5 \times 5}{6 \times 5} = \frac{25}{30}$$

$$\frac{9}{10} = \frac{9 \times 3}{10 \times 3} = \frac{27}{30}$$

In later examples, where this procedure is taking place, the region of working will be highlighted within a dotted rectangle as it has been in these examples. Of course, this is not necessary outside this book.

## Comparing Fractions

*Examples*

- Which is bigger: $\frac{3}{5}$ or $\frac{2}{3}$ ?

Some children would say $^3/_5$, because there are more segments, whereas others would say $^2/_3$ because the segments are bigger. Even a picture of the folded-paper version leaves some doubt (Figure 11.3a).

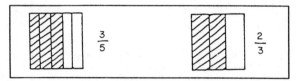

**Figure 11.3a**

Fractions can be compared best when their segments are the same size. This can be achieved by the procedure detailed in the previous section, which involves further folding, real, drawn, imagined or written. Again, the objective is a situation where both fractions have been through the same folding procedure. $^3/_5$ has been through fifthing. $^2/_3$ has been through thirding.

Therefore, $^3/_5$ now needs thirding and $^2/_3$ needs fifthing (Figure 11.3b).

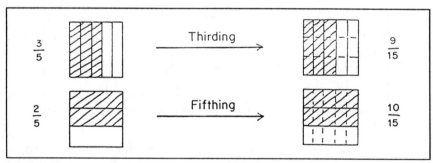

**Figure 11.3b**

The written version of this would be as shown in Figure 11.3c. Both the folded and written versions show $^2/_3$ to be bigger (by $^1/_{15}$).

$$\frac{3}{5} = \frac{3 \times 3}{5 \times 3} = \frac{9}{15}$$

$$\frac{2}{3} = \frac{2 \times 5}{3 \times 5} = \frac{10}{15}$$

**Figure 11.3c**

- Compare $^9/_{16}$ and $^5/_8$.

After considering how these fractions would be folded, it is evident that all that is now needed is for the 5/8 to undergo another halving process. Using only the written form:

$$\frac{9}{16} \quad = \quad \frac{9}{16}$$

$$\frac{5}{8} = \frac{5 \times 2}{8 \times 2} = \frac{10}{16}$$

which makes $\frac{5}{8}$ bigger (by $\frac{1}{16}$).

## Converting mixed fractions to top-heavy fractions

$2\frac{1}{4}$ is called a mixed fraction, because it has a whole number part and a fraction part. It is frequently necessary to convert all of this mixed fraction into segments (in this case quarters). Figure 11.4 shows the paper and written/spoken versions. The result is known as a top-heavy fraction for obvious reasons. The careful use of words in the written/spoken version is deliberate and necessary at first. This is because many children who have seen this work before remember incorrect methods. They remember a rule which says, 'Multiply something by something and add something', but unfortunately mix up their somethings. Until they understand why they are multiplying and adding, they are likely to produce $2 \times 1 + 4$ or $4 \times 1 + 2$ rather than $2 \times 4 + 1$.

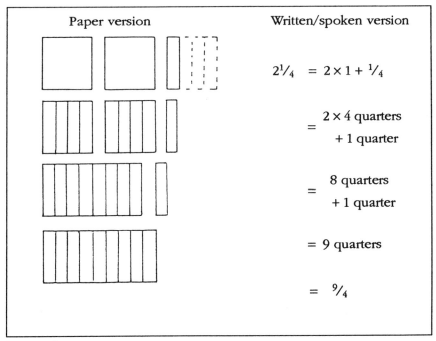

**Figure 11.4**

Subsequently they will perform the correct calculation in their heads, or write a variant of

$$2\frac{1}{4} = 2 \times \frac{4}{4} + \frac{1}{4}$$

$$= \frac{8}{4} + \frac{1}{4}$$

$$= \frac{9}{4}.$$

## Converting top-heavy fractions to mixed fractions

Top-heavy fractions have been called 'improper' fractions, a name which suggests it is undesirable to leave them in this form. They can be converted into mixed fractions as follows.

*Example*

- $\frac{14}{3}$

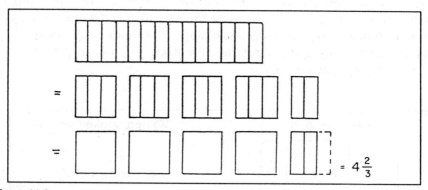

**Figure 11.5**

As the segments are thirds, they must be grouped in threes to form whole numbers (Figure 11.5). Any remainders will stay as thirds. The essential working is a division by three:

$$\begin{array}{r} 4r2 \\ 3\overline{)\,14} \end{array}$$

The results may be interpreted as follows:

| *Spoken version* | *Written version* |
|---|---|
| Fourteen thirds | $\frac{14}{3}$ |
| equals four times | |
| three thirds plus two thirds | $= 4 \times \frac{3}{3} + \frac{2}{3}$ |
| equals four whole | |
| numbers plus two thirds | $= 4 \times 1 + \frac{2}{3}$ |
| equals four and | |
| two thirds | $= 4\frac{2}{3}$ |

# Combining Fractions

## Vertical and horizontal presentation of fraction problems

We believe that a major cause of misunderstanding and confusion with fractions derives from the radical differences between the procedures used for addition and subtraction and those used for multiplication (and division). These differences are summarised in Table 11.1.

**Table 11.1**

| Addition/Subtraction | Multiplication |
|---|---|
| Addition and subtraction cannot take place until there are common denominators (i.e. equal segment sizes) | Multiplication can take place without common denominators |
| The denominators are neither added nor subtracted | The denominators (and numerators) are multiplied |
| Simplification is left to the end | Simplification is done as early as possible |
| Whole numbers are treated separately | Whole numbers are combined with fractions (to make mixed fractions) |

Paper folding is used as the (two-dimensional) model to illustrate the combining of fractions. This easy demonstration can be shown to dictate and therefore relate directly to the written algorithm. It simplifies each operation and provides a solution to the problem summarised in Table 11.1. It leads naturally to a vertical layout for addition and subtraction, which then contrasts with the horizontal presentation suggested for multiplication. Further advantages of this will be discussed later in this chapter.

The difficult concept of division of and, especially, division by fractions is also discussed later in the chapter. The 'normal' algorithms that are used to solve fraction-division problems must seem totally irrational and bizarre to many children (and adults). Some explanation is given, along with two methods, one vertical, one horizontal.

# Adding Fractions

This section starts by using paper folding to provide a concrete image of the operation. The explanation then moves to a more conceptual level in order to extend the child's performance and streamline his work. The initial descriptions progress from the easiest operation on fractions with the same denominator (segment size) to problems which involve mixed fractions.

## Fractions where the segments are the same size

*Example*

- $\frac{1}{5} + \frac{3}{5}$

Paper, written and spoken versions are given in Figure 11.6. The reference to a 'spoken version' introduces another two other senses, oral and aural, and emphasises that adding fifths to fifths produces fifths, that is, there is no change in segment size (or name), just as adding a number of marbles to another number of marbles still produces marbles. Thus examples of this type are used to establish that segments must be the same size before addition can proceed. You can judge how many examples of this type are needed to establish this fundamental precept.

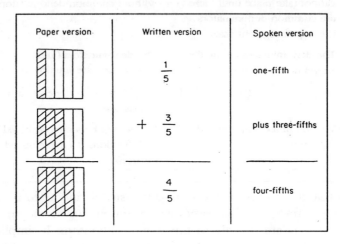

**Figure 11.6**

## Adding fractions where the segments are of different size

*Example*

- $\frac{1}{2} + \frac{2}{5}$

Again the different versions are given, in Figure 11.7. The paper-folding version signals a problem since the segments of the two pieces of paper in this type of problem are of different sizes. The spoken version confirms that like is not being added to like. Furthermore, if such an addition were to proceed, you could speculate about the problem with the child, 'What would be the segment size of the result?'.

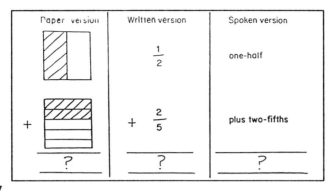

**Figure 11.7**

The child's attention should be focused on the segments, which are not the same size (or have the same name) and thus on the reason why addition cannot proceed without some modification to one or both of the segment names. The modification is to make the segments the same size (or give them the same name).

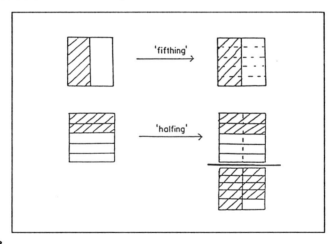

**Figure 11.8**

In this example the new segment size is tenths, because both halves and fifths can be renamed to this segment size (see Chapter 10). Both existing segments are folded again (Figure 11.8). The written version:

$$\frac{1}{2} = \frac{1 \times 5}{2 \times 5} = \frac{5}{10}$$

$$+\frac{2}{5} = \frac{2 \times 2}{5 \times 2} = \frac{4}{10}$$

$$\frac{9}{10}$$

follows the steps shown in Figure 11.8 with the paper and extends the method described in Chapter 10, which makes segments the same size.

## Adding more than two fractions

The same method, of making segment sizes the same, can be extended. Again the principle is to obtain the same segments for each fraction. Since more fractions are being added there is a likelihood of larger answers, possibly resulting in a top-heavy fraction.

*Example*

• $\quad {}^3/_4 \ + \ {}^1/_6 \ + \ {}^2/_3$

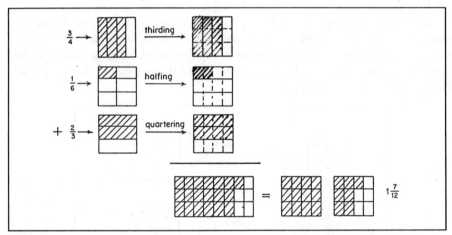

**Figure 11.9**

The common segment size is twelfths (Figure 11.9). The written version is:

$$\frac{3}{4} = \frac{3 \times 3}{4 \times 3} = \frac{9}{12}$$

$$\frac{1}{6} = \frac{1 \times 2}{6 \times 2} = \frac{2}{12}$$

$$+\frac{2}{3} = \frac{2 \times 4}{3 \times 4} = \frac{8}{12}$$

$$\frac{19}{12} = \frac{12}{12} + \frac{7}{12} = \frac{19}{12}$$

## Adding mixed fractions

*Mixed fractions with segments that are the same size*

The procedure is similar to the addition of simple fractions, but the child is learning to treat the whole numbers and fractions separately.

*Example*

• $2^{1}/_{5} + 3^{2}/_{5}$

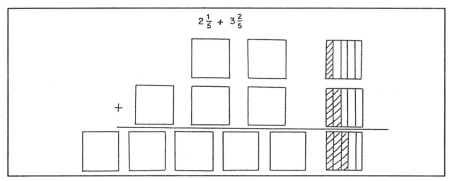

**Figure 11.10**

The folded-paper version (Figure 11.10) shows the answer clearly and also relates well to the written version:

| | | |
|---|---|---|
| $2^{1}/_{5}$ | | 21 |
| $3^{2}/_{5}$ | compare with | 32 |
| $5^{3}/_{5}$ | | 53 |

It demonstrates the need to deal separately with the whole numbers and the fractions in the same way that tens and units are dealt with separately in whole-number addition.

*Mixed fractions with different segment sizes*

Once again the child has to focus on the size of the segments and remember from the example above to deal with the whole numbers and fractions separately. Thus the exercise can be used to reinforce previously learnt skills.

*Example*

• $2^{1}/_{4} + 1^{2}/_{3}$

The written version is

$$2\,\frac{1}{4} = \frac{1 \times 3}{4 \times 3} \qquad\qquad = \frac{3}{12}$$

$$+1\,\frac{2}{3} = \frac{2 \times 2}{3 \times 2} = \frac{4}{6} = \frac{4 \times 2}{6 \times 2} \qquad = \frac{8}{12}$$

$$3 \qquad\qquad\qquad\qquad\qquad\qquad \frac{11}{12}$$

It would be simple to use paper folding to demonstrate the above steps, confirming the algorithm and the answer:

$$2\frac{1}{4} + 1\frac{2}{3} = 3\frac{11}{12}.$$

## Subtracting Fractions

The basic principle is the same as for addition. The child has to learn that the segments have to be the same size (same name) before subtraction can proceed. As with addition, a series of progressively more complex examples is given.

### Fractions where the segments are the same size

*Example*

- $\frac{3}{5} - \frac{1}{5}$

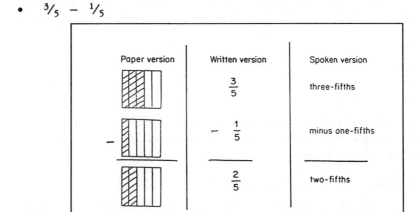

**Figure 11.11**

Paper, written and spoken versions are given in Figure 11.11. The spoken version confirms that the segments are the same size (have the same name) for the subtraction process.

### Fractions with different segment sizes

*Example*

- $\frac{4}{5} - \frac{2}{3}$

The paper version (Figure 11.12) shows that the problem is impossible to complete in this form (by showing different segment sizes). The spoken version confirms this because the segments have different names. The problem requires, as with addition, that the segments should be made the

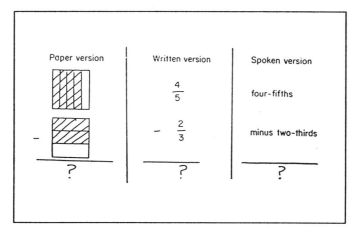

**Figure 11.12**

same size, in this case fifteenths. Again the concrete example of the paper folding focuses attention on the critical part of the algorithm, the need to work with segments which are the same size:

$$\frac{4}{5} = \frac{4 \times 3}{5 \times 3} = \frac{12}{15}$$

$$-\frac{2}{3} = \frac{2 \times 5}{3 \times 5} = \frac{10}{15}$$

$$\frac{2}{15}$$

## Subtracting mixed fractions

*Mixed fractions where the segments are the same size*

*Example*

- $3\frac{5}{9} - 2\frac{1}{9}$

The paper version is shown in Figure 11.13. The answer is quite clearly $1\frac{4}{9}$, and it is also clear that the whole numbers should be treated separately. The written version is as follows:

$$3\frac{5}{9} \qquad\qquad 35$$

$$- 2\frac{1}{9} \quad \text{compare with} \quad -21$$

$$\overline{1\frac{4}{9}} \qquad\qquad \overline{14}$$

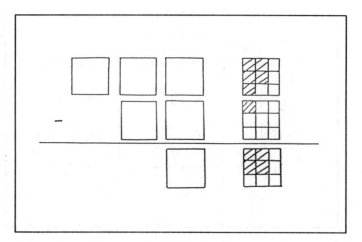

**Figure 11.13**

*Mixed fractions with different segment sizes*

Again the child has to focus on the segment sizes. The segments must be adjusted to be the same size (and to have the same name) and the whole numbers and parts must be dealt with separately. The child can use paper folding for all parts or just the fraction part of this problem. For the convenience of brevity only the written version is shown for this example:

- $5^5/_6 - 2^1/_4$

$$
\begin{array}{c|ccc}
5 & \dfrac{5}{6} = \dfrac{5 \times 2}{6 \times 2} & = & \dfrac{10}{12} \\[2ex]
-2 & \dfrac{1}{4} = \dfrac{1 \times 3}{4 \times 3} & = & \dfrac{3}{12} \\[2ex]
\hline
3 & & & \dfrac{7}{12}
\end{array}
$$

## Mixed fractions where a bigger fraction part is subtracted from a smaller fraction part

*Example*

- $4^1/_2 - 2^2/_3$

Since $^2/_3$ is bigger than $^1/_2$ the problem requires an adjustment not dissimilar to a whole-number subtraction such as $374 - 158$, where 8 is bigger than 4. The solution to the difficulty with fractions is very similar to that used with whole numbers. The child has to go to a whole number and con-

vert it to a fraction in the same way as a child doing a whole-number subtraction has to go to the tens column to obtain units.

Thus the algorithm is not another new, unrelated idea to learn. You are
showing the child the wide applicability of mathematical procedures. The
action of paper folding provides a concrete model for the algorithm and a
multisensory input to the memory. The paper-folding procedure also confirms for the child that $^2/_3$ is bigger than $^1/_2$. The paper version is given
in Figure 11.14 .

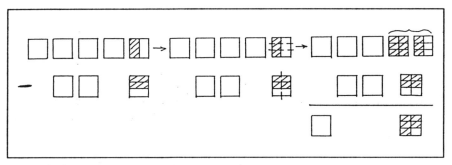

**Figure 11.14**

The written version is as follows:

$$4 \ ^1/_2 \ = 4 \ ^3/_6 \ = 3 \ \overbrace{^6/_6 \ \ ^3/_6}$$

$$-2 \ ^2/_3 \ = 2 \ ^4/_6 \ = 2 \quad \ ^4/_6$$

$$1 \quad \ ^5/_6$$

## Combined Additions and Subtractions

Both addition and subtraction of fractions require:

- segments of the same size (same name);

- whole numbers to be treated separately from parts.

Consequently, it is possible to perform both operations in the same calculation without a change of algorithm.

The child may need to use paper folding, but by now he may be able to
move straight to the written algorithm.

*Example*

- $2\frac{1}{8} + 3\frac{1}{2} - 1\frac{1}{4}$

$$
\begin{array}{rlcl}
2 & \dfrac{1}{8} & = & \dfrac{1}{8} \\[2ex]
+3 & \dfrac{1}{2} = \dfrac{1}{2} \times \dfrac{4}{4} & = & \dfrac{4}{8} \\[2ex]
-1 & \dfrac{1}{4} = \dfrac{1}{4} \times \dfrac{2}{2} & = & \dfrac{2}{8} \\[2ex]
\hline
4 & & & \dfrac{3}{8}
\end{array}
$$

It may be advantageous to show the child why the addition and subtraction of fractions have been presented in a vertical format. The following summarises the advantages.

**Advantages of the vertical layout for addition and subtraction of fractions**

1. It signals the need to make segment sizes the same.

2. There is less likelihood of adding or subtracting the denominators.

3. It allows room horizontally to change the segment sizes.

4. It lines up fractions and whole numbers separately and encourages the child to deal with them separately.

5. Numbers are added and subtracted vertically which is more familiar and easier for most children.

This layout is a well-established method of presentation in the USA.

# Multiplying by Fractions

The language of multiplication should be established first. As with percentages, the word 'of' is frequently used to mean multiply. For example $\frac{3}{4}$ of 8 means $\frac{3}{4} \times 8$. If the child needs to be convinced of this use, then reference back to whole number examples such as, 'How many sweets in 7 packets of 10?' or 'If a pen costs 20p, how much will I pay for 8 of them?' may help.

The language of fractions must also be revised. The child should be reminded that a fraction includes a hidden divide sign, so that $\frac{1}{3}$ means $1 \div 3$ and $\frac{4}{7}$ means $4 \div 7$.

The child has been told to focus on the bottom line of the fraction, the segment size (denominator). Now he needs to compare the relative value of the top and bottom lines to see if the fraction is bigger or smaller than 1. This is a necessary pre-skill for estimation work with fractions. Thus $3/8$ is smaller than 1 and $9/5$ is bigger than 1. (It is assumed, as with all suggestions, that you will expand on the examples given.)

## Estimation

The blunt estimate is to predict whether the answer to $a \times b$, where $b$ is a fraction, is smaller than $a$, has the same value as $a$, or is bigger than $a$. This can be explored via a sequence:

$5 \times 3 = 15$

$5 \times 2 = 10$

$5 \times 1 = 5$

$5 \times 2/5 = 2.$

1. When $b$ is bigger than 1, the product of $a \times b$ is bigger than $a$.

2. When $b$ is 1, the product of $a \times b$ is the same value as $a$.

3. When $b$ is smaller than 1, the product of $a \times b$ is smaller than $a$.

This latter conclusion can be discussed by considering the hidden division sign. For example, $15 \times 2/3$ is two operations: $15 \times 2$ $(=30)$, followed by $30 \div 3$; hence an answer of 10.

Thus an estimate can be made first on the simple observation as to the size of the fraction being bigger or smaller than one. The smaller the fraction (than 1), the smaller (relatively) the answer.

## Fraction times fraction

The multiplication of whole number by whole number (Chapter 8) used area as a model. Area is a two-dimensional model. The paper-folding model for fraction times fraction does the same.

Finding the fraction of a square of paper was explained earlier. Multiplication repeats the process in a second dimension. So one dimension represents $a$ and the other dimension represents $b$ in $a \times b$.

## Example 1

• $1/2 \times 1/3$

This multiplication is carried out by using a square of paper to find one half of one third of the square.

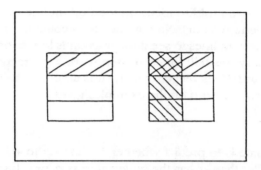

**Figure 11.15**

Figure 11.15 shows $\frac{1}{3}$ shaded. A second fold gives one half of this third. The part shaded twice is one half of one third. There are six segments in all, so one segment is $\frac{1}{6}$.

This was the method used earlier to find $\frac{1}{6}$, acknowledging the interrelationship among the fractions $\frac{1}{2}$, $\frac{1}{3}$ and $\frac{1}{6}$.

The application of two fraction operations to the same square has two major implications:

1. The change in segment size is seen to be inevitable. It should be obvious to the child that the answer will have a new segment size (and that it will be smaller).

2. The *horizontally* written layout of this multiplication reflects the difference of this operation and its model from that used for addition and subtraction.

The written form of the example above is

$$\frac{1}{2} \times \frac{1}{3} = \frac{1}{6}.$$

*Example 2*

- $\frac{2}{3}$ of $\frac{4}{5}$

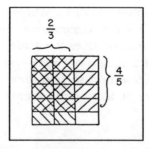

**Figure 11.16**

The square is folded into fifths in one direction and four of these fifths are shaded (Figure 11.16). The square is then folded into thirds in the opposite direction to give a grid with 15 segments, i.e. fifteenths. Two of the thirds are shaded (in the opposite direction) and the child should see the answer, $^8/_{15}$, shaded twice.

The concrete operation of folding and shading the square relates directly to the written form:

$$\frac{2}{3} \text{ of } \frac{4}{4} = \frac{2}{3} \times \frac{4}{5} = \frac{2 \times 4}{3 \times 5} = \frac{8}{15}.$$

The child is multiplying top and bottom parts of the fractions, which is easier to remember if the fractions are written side by side. The folding shows why 3 and 5 are multiplied together to make 15 segments and why 2 and 4 are multiplied together to give 8 of these segments.

### Example 3

- $^1/_2$ of $^4/_5$

This results in an answer which can be simplified or reduced. The paper-folding procedure is the same as in example 2, leading to an answer of $^4/_{10}$. Although this is not wrong, it would be more elegant to obtain $^2/_5$.

The written version may be used to explain cancelling before and after the multiplication. This offers an opportunity to remind the child that fractions are about division and that a fraction may have more than one 'name'.

### Fraction times whole number

*Example 1* (Figure 11.17a)

- $^1/_4$ of 1

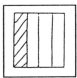

**Figure 11.17a**

*Example 2* (Figure 11.17b)

- $^1/_4$ of 3

The child should see that 1/4 of 3 is 1/4 three 'times', relating 'times' and 'of' once again. The written version relates exactly to fraction times fraction if 3 is written as 3/1:

$$\frac{1}{4} \text{ of } 3 = \frac{1}{4} \times \frac{3}{1} = \frac{1 \times 3}{4 \times 1} = \frac{3}{4}.$$

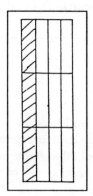

**Figure 11.17b**

*Example 3* (Figure 11.17c)

- $^2/_5$ of 2

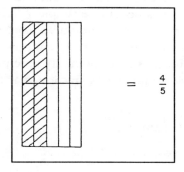

**Figure 11.17c**

The written version is

$$\frac{2}{5} \text{ of } 2 = \frac{2}{5} \times \frac{2}{1} = \frac{2 \times 2}{5 \times 1} = \frac{4}{5}.$$

# Multiplying Mixed Fractions

*Example*

- $3^1/_2 \times 2^1/_4$

The most probable error in this type of calculation arises when the child separates the fractions from the whole numbers, following an addition algorithm, and simply multiplies $3 \times 2$ and $^1/_2 \times ^1/_4$.

A consistent application of the area model for multiplication, $[(a+b) \times (c+d)]$, shows the need for four separate multiplications (see Chapter 8).

$3\frac{1}{2} \times 2\frac{1}{4}$ gives four areas, $A$, $B$, $C$ and $D$ (Figure 11.18).

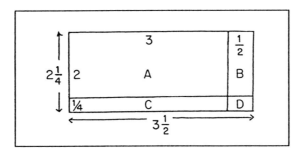

**Figure 11.18**

$A$ is $3 \times 2 = 6$ (which provides a simple estimate);

$B$ is $2 \times \frac{1}{2} = 1$;

$C$ is $3 \times \frac{1}{4} = \frac{3}{4} = \frac{6}{8}$;

$D$ is $\frac{1}{2} \times \frac{1}{4} = \frac{1}{8}$;

Total $= 7\frac{7}{8}$.

Although this provides a method consistent with that used for two digit times two digit whole-number multiplications, it is somewhat complex for fractions, so a procedure that is usually less open to errors is recommended. The mixed fractions are converted to top-heavy fractions, which can then be multiplied together as for simple fractions:

$$3\frac{1}{2} \times 2\frac{1}{4} = \frac{7}{2} \times \frac{9}{4} = \frac{7 \times 9}{2 \times 4} = \frac{63}{8} = 7\frac{7}{8}.$$

A new diagram can be drawn to illustrate this written method (Figure 11.19). This rectangle shows there are halves (seven of them) and that there are fourths (nine of them). The unit square shows the answer will be in eighths and the $7 \times 9$ grid shows there are 63 of these eighths. With these larger numbers there is more encouragement to cancel prior to multiplication.

*Example*

- $2\frac{2}{3} \times 2\frac{1}{10}$

$$2\frac{2}{3} \times 2\frac{1}{10} = \frac{8}{3} \times \frac{21}{10} = \frac{\overset{4}{8} \times \overset{7}{21}}{\underset{1}{3} \times \underset{5}{10}} = \frac{28}{5} = 5\frac{3}{5}.$$

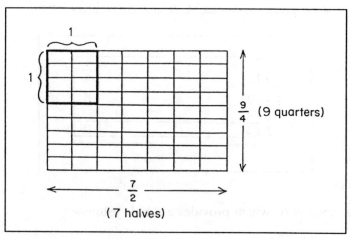

**Figure 11.19**

## The advantages of a horizontal layout for multiplication

1. It prompts the child to multiply the top numbers together and then to multiply the denominators together.

2. It encourages simplifying (cancelling) at the beginning.

3. There is less temptation to treat whole numbers in isolation.

4. It distinguishes between addition/subtraction and multiplication.

The advantages of different presentations for addition/subtraction and multiplication are best illustrated with an example which combines addition and multiplication.

*Example*

- $3\frac{1}{2} \times 1\frac{1}{2} + 1\frac{2}{3} \times 2\frac{1}{5}$

$$3\frac{1}{2} \times 1\frac{1}{2} = \frac{7}{2} \times \frac{3}{2} = \frac{7 \times 3}{2 \times 2} = \frac{21}{4} \qquad = \qquad 5 \quad \frac{1}{4} = \frac{3}{12}$$

$$+ \; 1\frac{2}{3} \times 2\frac{1}{5} = \frac{5^{1}}{3} \times \frac{11}{\cancel{5}_{1}} = \frac{1 \times 11}{3 \times 1} = \frac{11}{3} = \qquad 3 \quad \frac{2}{3} = \frac{8}{12}$$

$$\underline{\phantom{8}} \qquad \frac{11}{12}$$

$$8$$

multiplication $\longrightarrow$

addition

Many children will want to begin by inappropriate separation of the portions of the problem. You should encourage the child to read the problem and analyse its demands. The layout shown presents the problem clearly and logically.

The structured layout for the operations has extra advantages in this type of problem. It also follows the rules for the order of operations BOMDAS (Brackets Of Multiply Divide Add Subtract), where multiplication precedes addition.

## Dividing with Fractions

### Estimation

As with multiplication by fractions, division requires some development of number concepts. An estimate of an answer is a useful way of starting this work.

A sequence of divisions may be used to introduce the child to the concept (Ashcroft and Chinn, 1992):

$$20 \div 10 = 2$$

$$20 \div 5 \ = 4$$

$$20 \div 2 \ = 10$$

$$20 \div 1 \ = 20$$

$$20 \div \tfrac{1}{2} = 40.$$

Again this is focusing on whether the answer is bigger, the same or smaller than the original number.

In addition it may help the child to learn to rephrase the question, a strategy that has quite extensive value. Thus $20 \div \tfrac{1}{2}$ becomes 'How many halves in 20?'. You can develop this interpretation by using manipulative materials such as Cuisenaire rods, paper (folding), money, etc. For example, a square of paper may be folded to make two halves, followed by the question 'How many halves in one?'. It can be halved again, leading to the question 'How many quarters in one?'. The process can be continued through $\tfrac{1}{8}$, $\tfrac{1}{16}$, $\tfrac{1}{32}$ to show the answer becoming bigger as the fraction becomes smaller.

Thus the estimate is based on the relative value of the answer to the size of the initial number, as with multiplication: is it bigger, the same or smaller?

## Division by fractions

Two methods are described here. The first deals with simple examples and establishes a concrete image for this difficult concept. It is harder to explain the second method in this way, but it is the expedient way for those who progress to algebra.

The first method is set out vertically whereas the second method is presented horizontally (it being more akin to multiplication).

## Division by making the segments the same size

*Example*

- $^7/_{10} \div ^1/_{10}$

The spoken version of this problem needs a flexibility of mathematical vocabulary again. It could be read as 'Seven tenths divided by one tenth', but the child is more likely to understand 'How many tenths in seven tenths?'. Again the ability to rephrase a question can take the child a long way towards the answer of seven.

*Example*

- $^3/_4 \div ^1/_8$

The use of the same spoken version leads to 'How many (one) eighths in three quarters?'. This makes about as much sense as 'How many cars in a pencil?'. However, the alternative interpretation 'Divide three quarters into eighths' indicates more positively that the segment sizes should be made the same. So the first step is to make the segment sizes the same. Figure 11.20 shows the paper, written and spoken versions.

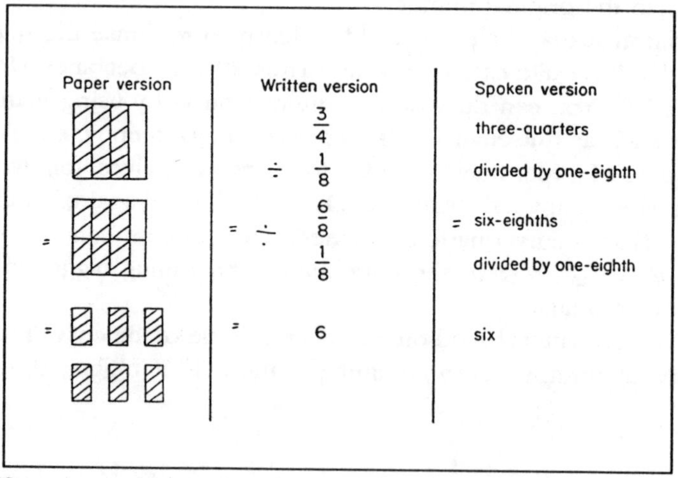

| Paper version | Written version | Spoken version |
|---|---|---|
| | $\dfrac{3}{4}$ | three-quarters |
| | $\div \dfrac{1}{8}$ | divided by one-eighth |
| = | $= \div \dfrac{6}{8}$ | = six-eighths |
| | $\dfrac{1}{8}$ | divided by one-eighth |
| = | = 6 | six |

**Figure 11.20**

*Example*

• $\frac{3}{5}$ + $\frac{7}{10}$

This is shown in the written version only:

$$\frac{3}{5} = \frac{6}{10}$$

$$+\frac{7}{10} = \frac{7}{10}$$

$$= \frac{6}{7}$$

## Examples with mixed fractions

The initial step of the method advocated is to convert the mixed fraction into a top-heavy fraction.

*Example*

• $3\frac{3}{4}$ + $\frac{3}{4}$

Since the segments are already the same the division proceeds immediately. The three versions are shown in Figure 11.21. The question is interpreted and illustrated as, 'How many groups of 3 (quarters) in 15 (quarters)?'.

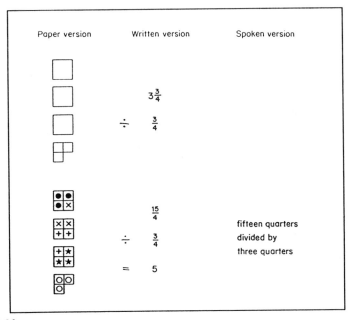

**Figure 11.21**

*Example*

• $5^2/_3 + 2^1/_2$

This is shown in written version only, because, by now the child should have a well established model of fractions:

$$5^2/_3 \quad = \frac{17}{3} = \frac{17 \times 2}{3 \times 2} = \frac{34}{6}$$

$$+ \; 2^1/_2 \quad = \frac{5}{2} = \frac{5 \times 2}{2 \times 3} = \frac{15}{6}$$

$$\frac{34}{15} = 2^4/_{15}$$

## Dividing fractions by inverse multiplication

This method is quicker, but asks the child to remember a seemingly inexplicable rule. So $4 + \frac{2}{3}$ is calculated as $4 \times \frac{3}{2}$. Some children will be happy enough to accept the explanation (rationalisation) that since multiplication is the opposite of division then there is a need to do an opposite thing with the fraction, that is, to turn it upside down.

An explanation for the algorithm can be developed for the child by a series of paper-folding exercises.

1.  $1 + \frac{1}{3}$

By definition, one whole number divided into thirds gives 3 (Figure 11.22a).

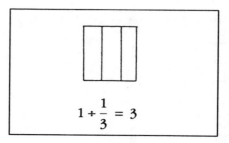

$$1 + \frac{1}{3} = 3$$

**Figure 11.22a**

2.  $4 \div \frac{1}{3}$

Four whole numbers divided into thirds will give 4 x 3 = 12 (Figure 11.22b).

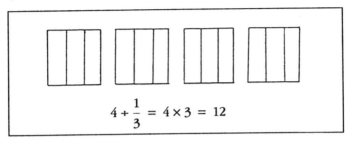

$$4 + \frac{1}{3} = 4 \times 3 = 12$$

**Figure 11.22b**

3.  $4 \div \frac{2}{3}$

4 divided into groups of two thirds will give (Figure 11.22c):

$4 \times 3 \div 2$     or     $4 \times 3$     or     6.

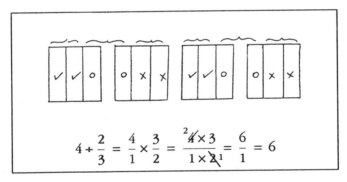

$$4 + \frac{2}{3} = \frac{4}{1} \times \frac{3}{2} = \frac{\overset{2}{4} \times 3}{1 \times \underset{1}{2}} = \frac{6}{1} = 6$$

**Figure 11.22c**

Since $\frac{2}{3}$ is twice as big as $\frac{1}{3}$, then the child should expect the answer to be half that of the previous example, that is, the previous answer has to be divided by 2. However you choose to justify the rule, it remains a case of inverting the fraction, then multiplying:

$$y \div \frac{a}{b} = y \times \frac{b}{a}.$$

# Chapter 12
# Decimals

## Introduction

It is the very great importance of the decimal point which engenders puns such as 'What's the point?' and visual jokes suggesting 'It's only a little dot'. Indeed, it is mainly the necessity to manoeuvre the decimal point into its correct position that differentiates decimal calculations from whole-number calculations. Apart from the decimal point, the processes of addition, subtraction, multiplication and division are identical to those covered for whole numbers in Chapters 7 and 8. The decimal point adds another 'dimension' to place value, and another potential source of errors.

It will be evident from the other chapters in this book that we are wary of teaching dyslexic children too many rules, because they are likely to forget or confuse them. However, this situation is an exception, largely because the rules for positioning the decimal point, once properly justified and established, are simple enough to make alternative procedures seem clumsy and pedantic. Indeed, ultimately, for all except multiplication, the rules boil down to keeping the decimal points under each other in a vertical line. Thus using a rule becomes pragmatically the best route.

## Addition and Subtraction

### Addition

Common errors tend to be due to misalignment of the decimal point – that is, incorrectly lining up the place values of the numbers involved (Ashlock, 1981). Such errors as

$$1.23 + 5 \quad \text{becoming} \quad \begin{array}{r} 1.23 \\ + 5 \\ \hline 1.28 \end{array}$$

and

$$0.09 + 0.5 \text{ becoming} \qquad \begin{array}{r} 0.09 \\ + 0.5 \\ \hline 0.14 \end{array}$$

demonstrate confusion over the positioning of the numbers in their columns and consequently of the decimal point. Reinstating column headings can help, but the tendency persists to line up the numbers from the right, irrespective of place value.

The correct process can be illustrated by using Dienes base-ten blocks or similar apparatus, but more effective help is usually achieved with the use of money. For example, children who begin by adding £1.23 + £5 with coins will rarely try to add the 5 and the 3, as in the written version above. Those children still tempted to do this usually respond to the suggestion that £5 may be written as £5.00, writing the .00 because it has no pennies, and so the written version becomes:

$$\begin{array}{r} £1.23 \\ + £5.00 \\ \hline £\,6.23 \end{array}$$

If written examples are linked, with the child handling the equivalent money, generally it becomes clear that pounds are added to pounds, pennies are added to pennies, and so on. The child can be led to write them under each other, which automatically puts the decimal points (separating the pounds and pennies) under each other. This gives the child a focus so that the other example from above can be presented as £0.09 + £0.5 (0) and written as:

$$\begin{array}{r} £0.0\ \ 9 \\ + £0.5\,(0) \\ \hline £0.5\ \ 9 \end{array}$$

Money provides the concrete memory hook for the child.

Another common error with decimal addition is shown below:

$$3.97 + 1.04 \text{ becomes} \qquad \begin{array}{r} ^{1} \\ 3.97 \\ + 1.04 \\ \hline 4.101 \end{array}$$

A child who produces this error has been content to carry a 1 from the hundredths to the tenths column, but is unwilling to carry a 1 from the tenths to the units column, which requires him to cross over the decimal point. There is a lack of understanding here that the decimal columns are simply an extension of the whole number columns, that they are related in the same way (increasing and decreasing in powers of ten) and that they must follow the same rules. This problem was anticipated in Chapter 10, where the issue was clarified by the use of decimal number sequences. A demonstration with money can be used to provide further reinforcement. The example above can be viewed as £3.97 + £1.04 and written

$$
\begin{array}{r}
{\scriptstyle 1\ 1} \\
£3.97 \\
+£1.04 \\
\hline
£\ 5.01
\end{array}
$$

Thus 7 + 4 is 11 pence, which is changed (traded) for a single ten pence, carried to the ten-pence column, and a one pence which is retained as the answer in the unit-pence column. Similarly, in the ten-pence column, the carried 1 is added to the 9 and 0 to give 10 lots of ten pence. These can be traded for £1, which is carried into the pounds column.

## Subtraction

Subtraction of decimal numbers presents children with virtually the same problems as addition. For example, 24.38 − 0.6 might generate the error

$$
\begin{array}{r}
24.38 \\
-0.6 \\
\hline
24.32
\end{array}
$$

Here the tendency to line up numbers from the right regardless of place value is compounded by the fact that the 6 is easier to subtract from 8 than 3. The solution to this problem is, as for addition, to line up the decimal points. Again the best manipulative material to illustrate and develop this procedure is money.

Another common error pattern is illustrated by the example 48.5 − 2.36. This tends to generate two types of error:

1.  Lining up from the right

$$
\begin{array}{r}
{\scriptstyle 7\ 1} \\
4\!\!\not{8}.5 \\
-2.36 \\
\hline
24.9
\end{array}
\quad \text{(or 2.49 and sometimes 2.4.9).}
$$

2. Setting up correctly, but

$$
\begin{array}{r}
48.5 \\
-2.36 \\
\hline 6
\end{array}
$$

The 6 is just transferred (effectively added) to the answer line, before the rest of the calculation is completed correctly.

$$
\begin{array}{r}
48.5 \\
-2.36 \\
\hline 46.26
\end{array}
$$

The use of an optional zero to 'square off' the calculation reminds the child that the 6 has to be subtracted, and gives him something to subtract from.

$$
\begin{array}{r}
48.50 \\
-2.36 \\
\hline
\end{array}
\qquad \text{then} \qquad
\begin{array}{r}
{}^{4}\!{}^{1} \\
48.\!\cancel{5}0 \\
-2.36 \\
\hline 46.14
\end{array}
$$

This can be practised with coins and place-value columns.

Errors in the addition and subtraction of decimals can be reduced through the policy of instilling into children the universal need to preview and review a question – to absorb some meaning and value for the numbers and produce an estimate – then check their answers against the estimate. This is likely to reduce the incidence of misalignment errors. Mention must also be made here of Ann Henderson's (1989) giant decimal point as another way of focusing attention on the all-important decimal point.

# Multiplication and Division by Powers of 10

### Multiplication by 10

As with so much work in mathematics, place value is important here, so a review of the topic may be an advisable precursor to the next work.

Confronted by the question $4.62 \times 10$, if the child can remember that $4 \times 10 = 40$ then this can help to lead him to see that $4.62 \times 10$ (4 and a bit times 10) should be forty-something. Alternatively, $4.62 \times 10$ can be interpreted as 10 lots of 4.62 and can be evaluated the 'long' way (as an addition):

$$
\begin{array}{r}
4.62 \\
4.62 \\
4.62 \\
4.62 \\
4.62 \\
4.62 \\
4.62 \\
4.62 \\
+\,4.62 \\
\hline
46.20
\end{array}
$$

Many children will notice that the figures 4, 6 and 2 have not changed, as might be expected in a multiplication; nor has their order. (This observation is, of course, an extension of the 10-times table pattern.) The numbers have moved along *one* place, so that each number is now ten times bigger. Most children can appreciate this pattern when it is pointed out to them. Base-ten blocks or money can be used for manipulative work.

As always, a multiplication is more efficient, quicker and less prone to error than the repeated addition of ten numbers.

The pattern can also be shown by considering each of the figures separately, using base-ten blocks, money or fractions to illustrate the procedure.

| 10 | 1 | $^1/_{10}$ | $^1/_{100}$ | | | | | 10 | 1 | $^1/_{10}$ |
|----|---|------------|-------------|---|---|---|---|----|---|-----------|
|    |   | (0)        | 2           | $\times 10 = ^2/_{100}$ $\times 10 = ^{20}/_{100} = ^2/_{10} =$ | | | |    |   | 2 |
|    |   | 6          |             | $\times 10 = ^6/_{10}$ $\times 10 =$ | | $^{60}/_{10} =$ | |    | 6 | |
| 4  |   |            |             | $\times 10 =$ | | | | 4 | 0 | |
| 4  | 6 | 2          |             | | | | | 4 | 6 | 2 |

| £1 | 10p | 1p | | | | £10 | £1 | 10p |
|----|-----|----|---|---|---|-----|----|-----|
|    | 0   | 2  | $\times 10 = 20p = 2 \times 10p =$ | | |     |    | 2 |
|    | 6   | (0)| $\times 10 = 60p \times 10 = £6 =$ | | |     | 6  | |
| 4  |     |    | $\times 10 =$ | £40 $=$ | | 4 | 0 | |
| 4  | 6   | 2  | | | | 4 | 6 | 2 |

When the pattern is written as $4.62 \times 10 = 46.2$, some children will imagine that the decimal point has moved rather than the figures. Whilst this is strictly incorrect, it is a simplification, the value of which can out-weigh its disadvantages and it is often the only way some children can remember the rule. In reality, the figures and the decimal point both move, relative to each other.

## Multiplication by 100

There are children who will be able to predict the effect of multiplying by 100 and they will conclude that the figures (or the decimal point) will move two places.

As with multiplying by 10, an example which relates to known facts can provide early understanding of the operation, as well as a valuable estimation procedure (useful also when calculators are used). For example, if it is known that $2 \times 100 = 200$, then $2.375 \times 100$ (which is 2 and a bit times 100) should be expected to be two hundred and a bit. Finally, if the digits are not to change, then the two hundred and a bit must be 237.5. This result can alternatively be justified by treating $\times 100$ as $\times 10 \times 10$ in two stages (compare to $\times 4$ as $\times 2 \times 2$ in Chapter 6), and by using the same manipulative materials used for $\times 10$:

$$2.375 \times 100$$
$$= 2.375 \times 10 \times 10$$
$$= 23.75 \times 10$$
$$= 237.5.$$

## Multiplication by 1000

At about this stage, children will usually see the pattern that the number of zeros in the multiplier dictates the number of places moved:

multiplying by 10          causes a movement of 1 place

multiplying by 100          causes a movement of 2 places,      so

multiplying by 1000          will cause a movement of 3 places.

For example, $27.1875 \times 1000 = 27187.5$. For justification, $\times 1000$ is equivalent to $\times 10 \times 10 \times 10$. The same manipulative materials may be used.

## Multiplication by other powers of 10

The pattern can simply be extended, using similar arguments, illustrations and materials.

## Division by 10

The initial goal is to show that division by 10 is the opposite of multiplication by 10. The answer becomes ten times smaller rather than ten times bigger. The topic could be introduced with money or base-ten blocks and the child being asked to show coins or blocks which are ten times bigger or ten times smaller. The answers are written on place-value paper. For example, 3p × 10 becomes 30p and conversely 30p ÷ 10 becomes 3p. The movement of the numbers is demonstrated by their places on the paper. A good demonstration of the required rule depends on the argument that a division by 10 and a multiplication by 10 will cancel each other out, because they are opposites:

$$so \quad \begin{array}{l} 37.63 \times 10 \div 10 = 37.63 \\ 376.3 \quad \div 10 = 37.63. \end{array}$$

The final line above shows that division by 10 causes a movement of one place. However, the movement is in the opposite direction to that caused by a multiplication by 10.

## Direction of movement

A decision about convention is now needed, concerning how to describe the direction of a movement. Referring to the direction as left or right would be ambiguous, because if the figures move left, the decimal point moves right, and vice versa. Furthermore, terms such as left and right, forwards and backwards, in front and behind are all likely to confuse dyslexics, with their laterality problems (Miles, 1983). We suggest that a safer and more meaningful practice is to describe the direction of movement in accordance with whether the answer is bigger or smaller than the original number.

- Multiplication by powers of 10 produces answers which are bigger than the original number.

- Division by powers of 10 produces answers which are smaller than the original number.

This convention encourages overviews, estimates and reviews.

## Division by 100, 1000 and other powers of 10

Divisions follow the same pattern as multiplications, in that the number of zeros in the divisor dictates the number of places moved (now in a direction which produces smaller answers).

- Dividing by 10 causes a movement of 1 place,     so

- Dividing by 100 causes a movement of 2 places

- Dividing by 1000 causes a movement of 3 places, etc.

This work can be justified, if necessary, by arranging divisions as repeated divisions by 10, or as reverse multiplications.

*Examples*

$$346.2 \div 100 = 3.462$$
$$1872.3 \div 1000 = 1.8732$$
$$23.721 \div 10000 = 0.0023721.$$

The last example illustrates the need to insert leading zeros, and the need to explain this to a child. Again there is the importance of using and appreciating place value.

**Rationalisation (1)**

It is worth anticipating children's potential problems with trying to apply these procedures to whole numbers – only decimal numbers have been used so far in this chapter. Whole numbers do not display a decimal point, so three is written as 3 and not 3.0. Many calculators will change an entry of 3.0 to 3 as soon as an operation key is pressed. Children tend to simplify multiplication and division of whole numbers by powers of 10 into a process of gaining or losing zeros. For example,

$$2 \times 10 = 2\underline{0}$$
$$3000 \div 1000 = 3\cancel{0}\cancel{0}\cancel{0} = 3.$$

It is important that children do not see the treatment of whole numbers and decimals as two different processes. The two situations can be rationalised by treating whole number examples as decimal examples:

$$2 \times 10 = 2.(0) \times 10 = 20(.) ;$$

here the digits and the decimal point have moved one place in a direction to make the answer bigger.

$$3000 \div 1000 = 3000.(0) \div 1000 = 3.(0000) ;$$

here there is a movement of three places to make the answer smaller.

Not only does this rationalise *all* multiplications and divisions by powers of 10, but these previously understood examples reinforce understanding of the new decimal work. Thus in $2 \times 10 = 20$ the digits and the decimal point *do* move one place.

## Multiplication of decimals by decimals

There is an expectation, rightly encouraged previously in this chapter, that multiplying a number will produce an answer which is bigger than the original number. This has been true for powers of 10. However, for the example $0.6 \times 0.8$ this will not be the case (see Rationalisation (2)). Consequently, such examples are very difficult for children still in the earlier stages to answer correctly, unless they apply the proper rule, backed up by estimating skills based on good number concept.

Establishment of the rule can begin using the area model (Figure 12.1) for multiplication, as in other chapters of this book. Within the unit square shown in the figure, the required answer is shown by the area of the shaded rectangle. The small squares, each $^1/_{100}$, show the answer to be $^{48}/_{100}$ or 0.48, which is less than either of the original numbers, 0.6(0) and 0.8(0). Of course this is because the answer represents part of a part.

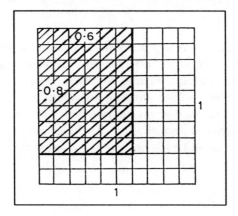

**Figure 12.1**

With or without the area model shown in Figure 12.1, the rule is best presented through fractions (Chapter 10 deliberately interrelated fractions, decimals and percentages), so $0.6 \times 0.8$ becomes:

$$\frac{6}{10} \times \frac{8}{10} = \frac{48}{100} = 0.48.$$

In this example, the decimal places for 0.6 and 0.8 are treated as tenths. The tenths accumulate, by multiplication, into hundredths, so any rule for the decimal places must reflect this accumulation:

| | |
|---|---|
| 0.6 | 1 decimal place |
| × 0.8 | 1 decimal place |
| 0.48 | 2 decimal places |

The decimal points do *not* line up under each other. The rule for positioning the decimal point can be stated as follows: 'The number of decimal places in the answer is equal to the total number of decimal places in the numbers of the question.' The digits in the answer (48) are the result of multiplying together the numbers in the question (6 and 8), and are obtained independently of the decimal places. Therefore, the numbers in the answer and the position of the decimal point are two separate considerations.

*Examples*

$$
\begin{array}{ll}
\phantom{\times}\ \ 0.0003 & \text{4 decimal places} \\
\times\phantom{\ \ \ }0.02 & \text{2 decimal places} \\
\hline
\phantom{\times}\ \ 0.000006 & \text{6 decimal places} \\
\end{array}
$$

$$
\begin{array}{ll}
\phantom{\times\ }3.2 & \text{1 decimal place} \\
\times\ 0.05 & \text{2 decimal places} \\
\hline
\phantom{\times}0.160 & \text{3 decimal places} \\
\end{array}
$$

$$
\begin{array}{ll}
\phantom{\times\ \ }21.09 & \text{2 decimal places} \\
\times\phantom{\ \ }3 & \text{0 decimal places} \\
\hline
\phantom{\times}63.27 & \text{2 decimal places} \\
\end{array}
$$

The final example shows that multiplication of a decimal by a whole number does not increase the number of decimal places. Quoting a special example such as this too early may lead to the impression that the decimal points do line up. Taken with other examples, this is seen to occur only in the exceptional case of a whole number multiplier.

## Rationalisation (2)

In this chapter, it has been suggested that children are taught to expect a larger answer after multiplying by a power of ten, but a smaller answer after multiplying by a decimal. There is no ambiguity here, and the following explanation can be used to rationalise the situation, and also to encourage good estimation and checking strategy. Use is made of a sequence such as:

$$45 \times 100 \quad = 4500$$
$$45 \times 10 \quad = 450$$
$$45 \times 1 \quad = 45$$
$$45 \times 0.1 \quad = 4.5$$
$$45 \times 0.01 \quad = 0.45$$

The pivotal value of multiplier is 1, because any number times 1 remains unchanged. A multiplier bigger than 1 gives an answer bigger than the original number, whereas a multiplier less than 1 gives an answer less than the original number. This leads to the basic estimate/check procedure: 'If the multiplier is bigger than 1, expect the answer to be bigger, and if the multiplier is less than 1, expect the answer to be smaller.' The overview is, once again, an important ingredient of the procedure.

(An interesting side-track concerns children's gut estimation of questions like $0.4 \times 0.002$. Given the choice of the answer being:

- bigger than 0.4

- a middle value between 0.4 and 0.002

- smaller than 0.002

most choose the middle value. A discussion as to the correct answer helps children understand the concept of multiplication by numbers less than 1 and acts as a useful reference/guide for similar problems.)

## Division of Decimals

### Division by a whole number

This work builds on the work of Chapter 9, with the added dimension of a decimal point, so a comparison with a whole-number example is a good lead in. $81 \div 3$ is traditionally set out as

$$
\begin{array}{r}
27 \\
3 \overline{)\ 81} \\
60 \\
\hline
21 \\
21 \\
\hline
0
\end{array}
$$

A pre-estimate of $81.6 \div 3$ might be 'a little more than 27, but less than 30'. The calculation could then be presented as

```
          27.2
      3) 81.6
          60.0
          ────
          21.6
          21.0
          ────
           .6
           .6
          ───
            0
```

The result compares well with the pre-estimate. For division by a whole number, the decimal points line up with each other. This algorithm sets the model for other decimal divisions.

### Division by a decimal

A question such as $8.64 \div 2$ follows the procedure above, because it is a division by a whole number. The question $8.64 \div 0.2$ will often be set out (erroneously) in the same way, as follows:

```
            4.32
     0.2) 8.64
            8.
            ──
            .64
            .6
            ───
             4
             4
            ──
             0
```

Of course dividing by 0.2 should produce a different answer and thus will need a modification to the method for dividing by 2.

A rephrasing of the language of the question can help. Instead of 8.64 divided by 0.2, the question can be understood as 'How many 0.2's in 8.64?' or 'How many £0.20's in £8.64?' with the extra help of examining the value of 0.2(0) and of using money to set up the question. A pre-estimate is then unlikely to suggest anything like 4 for the answer.

For the written, exact version, a solution to the problem lies in modifying the question so that it becomes a division by a whole number. This can be explained using equivalent fractions: $8.64 \div 0.2$ may be written as

$$\frac{8.64}{0.2} = \frac{8.64 \times 10}{0.2 \times 10} = \frac{86.4}{2} \quad \text{or} \quad 86.4 \div 2 \,.$$

Multiplying the top and bottom of the fraction alters the division to $86.4 \div 2$, without changing the final result. The process can also be seen as matching movements of the decimal places. The goal is to manoeuvre the decimal places of both numbers until the dividing number is a whole number (in this case 2).

The division can then proceed as in earlier examples:

```
          43.2
     2) 86.4
        80.0
        ────
         6.4
         6.0
         ───
           4
           4
         ───
           0
```

### Further examples

- $0.695 \div 0.05$ becomes $69.5 \div 5$ (moving both numbers two places)

```
          13.9
     5) 69.5
        50.0
        ────
        19.5
        15.0
        ────
         4.5
         4.5
        ────
           0
```

- $13.2 \div 0.006$ becomes $13200 \div 6$ (moving both numbers three places), etc.

- $0.13 \div 0.8$ becomes $1.3 \div 8$ (moving both numbers one place)

```
      0.1625
 8) 1.3000
     .8
     .50
     .48
     20
     16
     40
     40
      0
```

Note that in the final example 1.3 was written as 1.3000. The extra zeros are optional (see Chapter 10) and do not affect the value, but help with the setting out of the question.

### Approximations/rounding

Sometimes it is desirable to give an approximate answer in round figures. For example, £8.29 might be described as 'nearly £8.30 (£8.3)', or 'about £8'.

- 8.29 is somewhere between 8.20 and 8.30. It is nearer to 8.30, because it is above the half-way position of 8.25. Therefore, rounded to 1 decimal place, 8.29 would be written as 8.3.

- 8.29 is somewhere between 8 and 9. It is nearer to 8, because it is below the half-way position of 8.50. Therefore, rounded to the nearest whole number, 8.29 would be written as 8.

Such separate judgements need not be made, when a general policy is agreed. Where practicable, a number line (Figure 12.2) shows quite clearly which approximation is nearer.

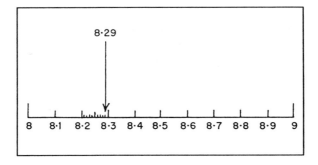

**Figure 12.2**

A numerical policy is more readily applicable, however. The accepted policy is demonstrated in Table 12.1 through rounding a complete set of numbers to 1 decimal place. The place to be retained is separated by a line from the place to be lost.

**Table 12.1**

|  |  |  |  | Nearer to | Rounded to |
|---|---|---|---|---|---|
| .60 | = | .6 | 0 | .60* | .6 |
| .61 | = | .6 | 1 | .60 | .6 |
| .62 | = | .6 | 2 | .60 | .6 |
| .63 | = | .6 | 3 | .60 | .6 |
| .64 | = | .6 | 4 | .60 | .6 |
| .65 | = | .6 | 5 | .70* | .7 |
| .66 | = | .6 | 6 | .70 | .7 |
| .67 | = | .6 | 7 | .70 | .7 |
| .68 | = | .6 | 8 | .70 | .7 |
| .69 | = | .6 | 9 | .70 | .7 |

It can be seen that:

1. when the place to be lost contains a 5 or more, the number retained is rounded up, by adding 1;

2. when the place to be lost contains a 4 or less, the number retained is rounded down, by adding 0.

This is the policy normally applied, because it is even-handed -- half of the numbers are rounded up, and half are rounded down. In fact it embodies the twin fallacies (see values with * in Table 12.1) that

- .60 needs rounding to .6, and

- .65 is nearer to .70 than .60.

Sometimes a division will produce an answer which is too long, and will have to be shortened, by rounding off excess places. Indeed, some divisions, such as 39.5 + 7 would carry on for ever. The early part of this calculation is shown:

```
        5.64285, etc
   7) 39.50000
      35
     ────
       4.5
       4.2
      ────
        30
        28
       ────
        20
        14
       ────
        60
        56
       ────
        40
        35
```

The answer to this division is now given in various approximations:

- 5.(64285 = 6 to the nearest whole number, because a 6 is rounded off;

- 5.6(4285 = 5.6 to 1 decimal place, because a 4 is rounded off;

- 5.642(85 = 5.643 to 3 decimal places, because an 8 is rounded off;

- 5.6428(5 = 5.6429 to 4 decimal places, because a 5 is rounded off.

Some decimals are particularly awkward to round. For example, approximating 9.999 to two decimal places. When rounding off the final 9, the 9 in the second decimal place must be rounded up, by adding 1. The likely problems here are avoided by actually carrying out an addition:

```
    9.99
   + 1
  ──────
   10.00
```

The act of rounding up has a knock-on effect for all the other figures. The two zeros after the decimal point must be retained – normally regarded as optional, they are needed here to give the approximation to the required number of decimal places.

Rounding must be performed in a single step, for accuracy. Rounding in stages can produce errors. For example,

6.247 = 6.2 correct to 1 place.

However, rounding in stages gives

6.247 = 6.25 correct to 2 places, then

6.25 = 6.3 which is wrong.

## Converting harder fractions to decimals

In this chapter, it is possible to cover the types of example, like $\frac{5}{9}$, which were beyond the scope of the methods used in Chapter 10. The diagrams in Figure 12.3 are intended to show that $\frac{5}{9}$ is the same as $5 \div 9$.

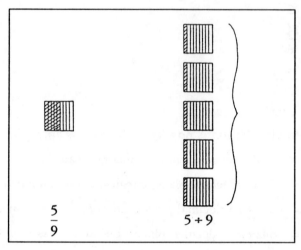

**Figure 12.3**

The conversion of $\frac{5}{9}$ to a decimal can now be achieved by performing $5 \div 9$ as a decimal division, and rounding the answer to, say, three decimal places. It will be necessary to work out four decimal places, so that the size of the fourth decimal place, and its consequent effect on the third decimal place, can be determined.

```
        0.5555, etc.
   9) 5.0000
      4.5
      ___
       50
       45
       __
        50
        45
        __
         50
         45
```

0.5555 = 0.556 correct to three decimal places.

$\frac{5}{9}$ = .556 correct to three decimal places.

This method of conversion works for any fraction, even the earlier easy examples. Furthermore, in Chapter 10, the conversion to a decimal of $\frac{7}{8}$ was seen to require some special knowledge. Now it can be carried out mechanically as 7 + 8 .

```
        0.875
   8 ) 7.000
       6.4
       ───
        60
        56
       ───
        40
        40
       ───
        00
       ──
```

$\frac{7}{8}$ is equivalent to the exact decimal .875.

## Summary

As outlined at the beginning of this chapter, the methods used to justify the rules for decimals would seem far too complicated for most children. Instead, once the rules are understood, it is much simpler to stick to them. The working involved with deriving the rules may be worth showing to some children just once, or it may be held in reserve by the teacher, in case of awkward questions.

The rules concerning the positioning of the decimal point summarise as follows:

1. For addition or subtraction, all the decimal points of the question and the answer line up vertically.

2. The same is true for a division, once it has been modified into a division by a whole number. This is achieved by moving the figures (or the decimal point) in both numbers by the same number of places, as appropriate.

3. The decimal points in a multiplication do not line up. The number of decimal places in the answer is given by the total number of decimal places in the question. The actual numbers can be multiplied together in the normal way.

4. Multiplication and division of decimals by 10, 100, 1000, etc. never change the figures – they merely move them. The number of places moved is dictated by the the number of zeros, whereas the direction of movement gives a bigger answer for multiplication, and a smaller answer for division.

Because addition, subtraction and division ultimately follow the same rule, some teachers prefer to teach them first, in the given order. Multiplication, the odd one out is then dealt with last.

Finally, and leaving out much of the detail, the policy for approximating reduces to:

• 5 or more means round up

• 4 or less means round down.

# Chapter 13
# Percentages

## Introduction

In Chapter 10 percentages were related to decimals and fractions, with emphasis on reference/key values such as 50% and 10%. In this chapter the work will be extended to all numbers, but those reference values will still be referred to for pre- and post-estimates. The key idea of this chapter is to provide a concrete image of percentages so that the formulae and algorithms have a memory base. The image should also instil an understanding of the concept of percentages. This is achieved by focusing on 100 and one. There is a consequence of this image, in that focusing on one leads to a division before a multiplication. This is in contradiction to BOMDAS, the normal order for operations, and could lead to compounding errors of earlier rounding/estimations of numbers. Despite this, we feel that the strong image given by the advocated method overcomes this disadvantage.

## An Image of Percentage

Since percentage relates to 100, then the image presented to the pupil should involve a clear demonstration of 100. Further it should demonstrate dividing the quantity up into 100 parts (thereby identifying one part). A clear method for this uses empty 35 mm film tubs, 100 of them arranged in a 10-by-10 square (Figure 13.1).

There are three types of percentage problem.

- Type 1 is 'What is $n$% of $N$?' (finding the percentage of a quantity).

- Type 2 is 'What percentage of $y$ is $x$?' (one quantity as a percentage of another).

- Type 3 is '$x$ is $n$% of which number?' (finding the original number).

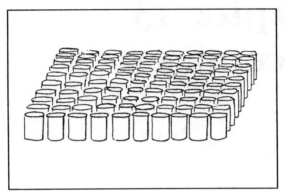

**Figure 13.1.** 100 film tubes

Each type is explained in turn.

### Type 1. What is *n*% of *N*?

An example can be used to show the tubs in use. The question is, 'What is 12% of 300?' An 'easy' question is used to set up the illustration and lead into more 'difficult' numbers.

300 (plastic) pence are used. The pence are divided up into the 100 tubs (evenly). One tub is examined and will contain three pence. You can discuss and explain that the tub represents one out of 100 tubs and that its contents represent $\frac{1}{100}$ of the 300 pence or 1% of the 300. The pupil is asked what two tubs represent and what is in the two tubs and then for three tubs, five tubs and ten tubs, at which stage the pupil can be referred back to 10% as equivalent to $\frac{1}{10}$ as a check. You can emphasise the process as dividing up into 100 (equal) parts to obtain 1 part (1%) and the use of this 1% to find 12% or any other percentage.

This demonstration relates directly to the written algorithm; 300 is divided by 100 and the result is multiplied by 12. This can be represented as a flow chart (Figure 13.2) or as an equation:

$$(300 \div 100) \times 12.$$

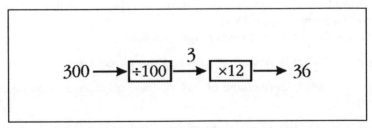

**Figure 13.2**

The work can be extended, depending on the age and ability of the pupil, to lead to the general formula for 'What is $n$% of $N$?', i.e. $(N/100)n$.

Other examples can be demonstrated and/or discussed, such as 8% of 60, where 60 is less than 100. So each tub gets less than 1 and (probably via some revision on dividing by 100 and obtaining decimals) or by using money and imagining £0.60 in each tub.

The algorithm is clearly related to the concrete image of first dividing up into 100 equal parts, followed by taking $n$ lots of these parts, i.e. a division followed by a multiplication.

### Type 2. 'What percentage of $y$ is $x$?'

This type of percentage is often presented as an examination-score type of question: If a pupil gets 46 out of 85 in his maths examination, what is his percentage mark? It is asking the pupil to convert $x/y$ into a percentage. The film tubs keep the image of 100 in the pupil's mind. The procedure then is to change $x/y$ into a decimal and to know that the resulting decimal represents the amount in one tub.

So, in the example above, 46 out of 85 becomes $46/85 = 0.5412$ which is 54.12%. This last step can be done by knowing that 0.5412 is the number in one tub and multiplying the decimal 0.5412 by 100 to find the number in 100 tubs, i.e. 100%.

This method uses the same image as for the first type of problem. The focus is on what is in one tub (1%) and then to multiply that value for 1% up to the required value, in this case 100%.

If we refer back to Chapter 10, the procedure could also be to change $x/y$ to an equivalent fraction with denominator 100. The pupil has to appreciate that a percentage is a fraction with a denominator of 100, where only the value of the numerator is quoted.

### Type 3. '$x$ is $n$% of which number?'

Again the focus is on 1%. So in an example such as '36 is 12% of which number?' the first operation is to calculate 1%, i.e what goes into one tub? The child is asked 'If there are 36 in 12 tubs, can you work out how many in one tub?'. This should result in an answer of three in each tub. The 100% is then a matter of multiplying three by 100, answer 300.

## Summary

The film tubs provide the image of 1% and 100% in a way that allows the algorithm to be related directly to the image/model. The child has to evaluate the data in each question and form a mental image of what goes into each tub in order to understand a difficult concept and procedure.

# Chapter 14
# Introducing
# Other Topics

## Introduction

Faced with a dyslexic pupil, who at a young age is experiencing great difficulty with mathematics, you may feel it best to persevere with the basics of numeracy until the pupil has mastered them. You may regard these basics as so fundamentally important that to proceed to other topics does not seem to represent the best use of time or effort. As time passes, however, and the pupil continues to experience the same difficulties, the temptation grows to concentrate even harder on a narrow range of activities. Such a situation can come to extend over a period of years, during which the dyslexic child is enduring constant failure and losing all confidence in himself and the learning process. The loss of confidence is a serious additional problem in a subject where confidence in performance is so important – mathematics is like walking a tight-rope, in the sense that if you think you are going to fall, then you will probably fall.

Varying the mathematical diet for such a pupil is a course of action which may have beneficial effects of three kinds.

1. It may provide him with a small amount of success and bring back some confidence.

2. Even more importantly, it may begin a process that gives him an alternative way of looking at the subject – a way around his problems when there may be no way through them. If building a wall can be used as a metaphor for the learning of mathematics, then the wall of a dyslexic child will have many bricks missing, parts of the subject he has not mastered. However, a wall can, of course, remain standing around a few gaps and, the wider the wall, the more missing bricks it can bridge and still provide support. Where the wall of a dyslexic child cannot be built directly upwards, it should be built across and then upwards, by widening his mathematical experience, especially at the foundation levels.

3. It may give him abilities, such as telling the time, which can be regarded as social or 'survival' skills (Copeland, 1984), the lack of which can be embarrassing for the child (or his parents).

It is possible to introduce other mathematical topics than number, in such a way that they reinforce the numerical work, rather than just adding to the load. This chapter begins with examples of short topics treated in this way, continues with an illustrative long topic, Time, and concludes with a discussion of some typical points of difficulty for dyslexics.

## Introducing Short Topics

*Example 1*

Addition in two digits can be illustrated by covering concurrently the combination of angles, like those shown in Figure 14.1a:

$$
\begin{array}{r}
25 \\
+\,50 \\
\hline
75 \\
\hline
\end{array}
$$

The idea of combining angles can be extended to the case where angles are represented by letters (Figure 14.1b).

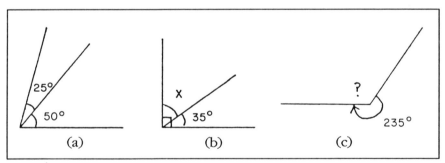

(a)  (b)  (c)

**Figure 14.1**

It involves very little extra difficulty for a child to add the angles in Figure 14.1b and obtain $x + 35$. It is also conceivable, at this stage, for him to form the equation $x + 35 = 90$, since the outer angle has been carefully chosen as a right angle.

*Example 2*

When children are practising subtraction of hundreds, tens and units, its application to an example such as that in Figure 14.1c can provide credibility and motivation:

$$\begin{array}{r} {}^{5}\cancel{3}{}^{1}\cancel{6}0 \\ -235 \\ \hline 125 \end{array}$$

## Example 3

Sometimes a carefully chosen example can help children to derive rules themselves, which means that they will understand them well, and remember them more easily. At a time when perimeter has been studied, Figure 14.2 could lead elsewhere.

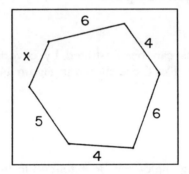

**Figure 14.2**

If the length of the perimeter is 28, prompted by the question: 'How would you find $x$?', many children would have no difficulty in concluding that the given sides should be added, and the total subtracted from 28. A written version of the problem and its solution:

$$x + 6 + 4 + 6 + 5 + 4 = 28$$
$$x + 25 = 28$$
$$x = 28 - 25$$
$$x = 3$$

indicates precisely how quite difficult equations should be solved, the rule being:

- Change the *side* – change the *sign*.

## Example 4

The problem:

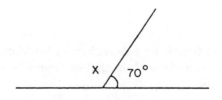

can be regarded as a spatial problem. The calculation of the missing angle can be performed numerically, as $180 - 70$, or interpreted algebraically in the form of the equation $x + 70 = 180$. Furthermore, if the problem was generalised as:

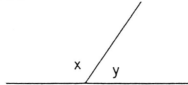

and the value of $x$ was allowed to vary, between 0 and 180, then the corresponding values of $y$ could be tabulated against it, as in Table 14.1, which shows all possible pairs of values for multiples of 20 and could be generalised into the relationship $y = 180 - x$. A graph of the values in the table (shown next to Table 14.1) would produce a backwards-sloping straight line (rare in itself at this level), which can be used to show every possible pair of values and thereby demonstrate the problem-solving power of graphs.

**Table 14.1**

| x | y |
| --- | --- |
| 0 | 180 |
| 20 | 160 |
| 40 | 140 |
| 60 | 120 |
| 80 | 100 |
| 100 | 80 |
| 120 | 60 |
| 140 | 40 |
| 160 | 20 |
| 180 | 0 |

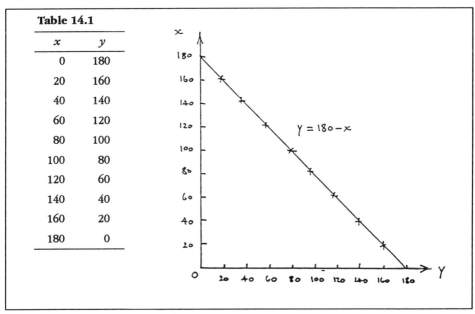

## Introducing Time

This section addresses two aspects of time, telling the time and simple problems with time. Although discussed here together, such a lengthy topic should almost certainly be taught in smaller, separate portions (see Chapter 15). The timing of the topic's introduction should also be considered carefully (see Chapter 15). Copeland has observed that some children at age ten are still not ready for a true understanding of time, so some of the work in this section may be too advanced for children who are slightly older than this, but whose learning difficulties have held them back.

Being unable to tell the time is a classic weakness for dyslexics. The advent of the digital watch has enabled more children to say the time, but it has not necessarily enabled them to have a concept of time. Being able to read a timetable or work out journey times are life skills and involve an understanding of the 24-hour clock. Concentrating on the two basic areas referred to in the previous paragraph covers the majority of needs without overcomplicating the issue.

Time involves the child in some new ideas, particularly working in new number bases: 12, 24 and 60. 'Traditional' time-telling involves not only adding time (as minutes and quarters) after the hour, but also counting down time to the next hour. The topic also uses some fraction work and a number line, but these too are different, since both are based on a circle (Figure 14.3).

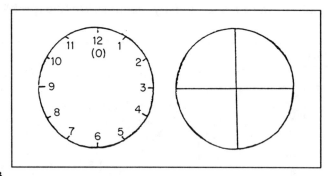

**Figure 14.3**

Thus the child has to adapt to these new demands and will probably adapt more successfully if the work is built on his existing knowledge and adjusted to this new framework. The new framework will be stronger if it is based, not on the digital clock or watch (which has the tempting advantage of being easy to read), but on the traditional, analogue clock. The clock face provides better memory hooks and a better understanding of the relative place of times, gives 12 a prominent place and can be used to develop more strategies for the child. A digital clock does not have these advantages.

### Setting the scene

The best visual aid is obviously a clock. Although cardboard 'play' clocks are cheap, a better demonstration is achievable with a real clock. A real clock has hands which are synchronised, so that as the minute hand moves round, the hour hand moves towards the next hour. This gives the child the image of time: seconds, minutes and hours all moving constantly onwards, each at its own pace. The clock face has 12 at the top, and 12, like 100 for percentages, is a critical number to remember.

As mentioned above, one of the teaching approaches advocated in this book is to start work from the child's interests and his existing knowledge base (a base that is usually bigger than he thinks, once some careful teasing out of facts and organisation has been accomplished). The initial approach described below is an illustration of this technique.

Starting with the assumption that the child must have had some experience of times, such as the time school finishes, the time a favourite television programme starts and so on, you can ask the child to say some times he knows, and you can write them down so that the child can see them on paper as well as on a clock. You may need to prompt with questions like: 'What time do get up to go to school/on a weekend?' Work of this kind concentrates on showing the child the need to identify hours and minutes for telling the time, without asking the child actually to tell the time.

Looking at material like the day's television programme times confirms this need and shows how times are presented. Again link this to the clock, with exercises that include asking the child to identify the hands and to show the number of minutes around the clock and the number of hours around the clock. The synchronised hour and minute hands can be used by the child to confirm that as the minute hand moves once around the clock, the hour hand moves steadily on to the next hour.

The combination of the material showing written times and observation of the clock can lead to a discussion of morning and a.m., evening and p.m. and the importance of 12 o'clock. Thus an understanding will develop of a day being two circuits of the clock, and therefore 24 hours. You can also stress again that time is continuous. (Another social-skill problem involving time is the dyslexic's tendency to confuse the names of meals and to say 'Good afternoon' or 'Good morning' at the wrong time of day. It may be useful to introduce these items into appropriate examples.)

The clock and the movement of the hands round and round show the continuous nature of time. It also shows that the minute hand can point to any number up to 60, and that 60 coincides with the 0 of the next circuit. Likewise, it shows that the hour hand can point to any number up to 12, and that 12 coincides with the 0 of the next circuit. You can show the child how the hour hand is half-way to the next hour when the minute hand is on 30 (half past). The clock face needs to be seen as a number line, but instead of going on and on like a linear number line, it circles back to zero every 60 seconds for the second hand, every 60 minutes for the minute hand and every 12 hours for the hour hand. (At this stage the 24-hour clock is held in abeyance.)

## Quarter past, half past and quarter to

These reference times can be fairly easily mastered. The clock face can be divided into a half (possibly using a cut-out circle) and the number of minutes in a half hour discussed. This leads on to quarters, again with paper folding.

This is an appropriate place to introduce the ideas of time past and time to, which form part of the the understanding of time as opposed to just saying the time (from a digital watch). (In the UK 'past' and 'to' are used; in the USA 'after' and 'before'.) The child is introduced to half being a change-over point. Up to the half the minutes are counted as time past, so the first quarter is 'quarter past'. The half is 'half past', but after this, time starts to look forwards towards the next hour, so the last quarter is 'quarter to' the next hour (Figure 14.4). (There is some similarity here to the work the child did in 'making change' – counting on the money to take him up to a pound or whatever.)

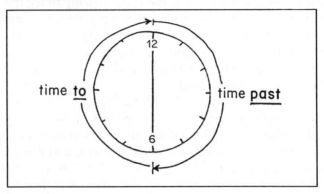

**Figure 14.4**

A rational explanation for the child is that you only refer to the nearest hour. After 30 minutes, the next hour is nearer. The position of the hour hand aids this explanation (Figure 14.5). (Other examples abound, such as the countdown for rockets, the number of shopping-days to Christmas and so on.)

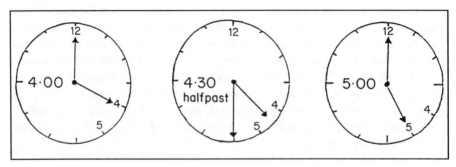

**Figure 14.5**

## Minutes past

There are 30 minutes which can be 'past' the hour. These are not numbered on the clock, but are grouped in 5's for each hour number; this acts as another reinforcement of the 5-times table. The quarter hour acts as a mid-way reference point of 15 minutes (Figure 14.6a).

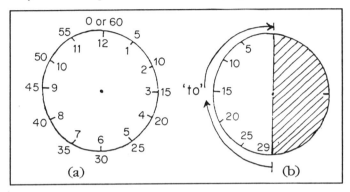

**Figure 14.6**

## Minutes to

There are 29 minutes which can be 'to' the hour, starting straight after the half (30) and counting down to the hour (0) (Figure 14.6b). Again they are grouped in 5's, working down through the mid-way reference point of 'quarter to' (15). The child must remember that as the minute hand gets closer to the next hour, the number of minutes left 'to' the hour gets less.

## Ante meridian (a.m.) and post meridian (p.m.)

With older children (aged, say, 12 or 13), a good problem is as follows. Here is a new form of addition. See if you can find how it works:

$6 + 2 = 8$

$7 + 4 = 11$

$8 + 7 = 3$

$10 + 8 = 6$       (10 a.m. to 12 noon, 12 noon to 6 p.m.)

$11 + 5 = ?$

This introduces the child to the concept of base 12 as a puzzle and focuses attention on the need to use a different base when adding hours. It also emphasises the importance of 12 as a finish/start point. The descriptive names of midday and midnight add to this image of 12 as special and help the child conceptualise a.m. and p.m.

## Time problems

The puzzle in the section above introduces time-gap problems, such as 'If I start a journey at 9 a.m. and travel for 10 hours, when do I arrive?'. If these are done without using the 24-hour clock, then two methods are available.

- Base-12 correction Add the times and subtract 12 (if necessary) to obtain the p.m. (or a.m.) time:

$$
\begin{array}{r}
9 \\
+\,10 \\
\hline
19
\end{array}
\qquad \text{then} \qquad
\begin{array}{r}
19 \\
-\,12 \\
\hline
7 \text{ p.m.}
\end{array}
$$

(This method is using the 24-hour clock without acknowledging it.)

- Go via 12 on the number circle (Figure 14.7).

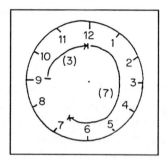

**Figure 14.7**

$12 - 9 = 3$ hours (before 12)

$10 - 3 = 7$ hours (after 12)

Total = 10 hours.

The same methods can be modified to deal with subtraction problems, such as: 'A woman works from 10 a.m. until 3 p.m. How long does she work?'

- Base-12 correction:

Add 12 to the *end* time (again the 24-hour clock adjustment):

$$
\begin{array}{r}
3 \\
+\,12 \\
\hline
15
\end{array}
$$

Subtract the *start* time:

$$\begin{array}{r} 15 \\ -10 \\ \hline 5 \end{array} \text{ hours}$$

- Go via 12 on the number circle (Figure 14.8).

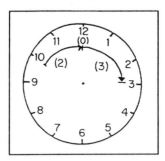

**Figure 14.8**

$$\begin{array}{r} 12 \\ -10 \\ \hline 2 \end{array} \quad \text{and} \quad \begin{array}{r} 3 \\ 0 \\ \hline 3 \end{array}$$

so

$$\begin{array}{r} 2 \\ +3 \\ \hline 5 \end{array}$$

## The 24-hour clock

The advent of the digital watch, digital clock and video recorder has familiarised children with the 24-hour clock. It is, therefore, less likely to be a revelation to many children. The clock face, the length of the day ($2 \times 12 = 24$) and the base-12 work above all acted as introductory material to this topic. It is not difficult to show a child how the 24-hour clock replaces the need for a.m. and p.m.

Conversion is via 12, which is added or subtracted according to the problem. It helps the child to have a reference time for use as a model to check if he has to add or subtract. This could be the end of school, say '4 p.m. as 16:00 hours' or a favourite television programme, '7:30 p.m. as 19:30 hours'.

It is strongly advised that times are never written with a point, as in 7.30, since this is likely to suggest that time works in decimal (base 10) and undermine much of what is contained elsewhere in this chapter. The colon, much used in digital displays, is a safe replacement, giving 7:30, the form used above.

*Examples*

- 5 p.m. as 24-hour time is $5 + 12 = 17:00$

- 19:00 hours is $19 - 12 = 7$ p.m.

A clock face with the 24-hour numbers added (Figure 14.9) helps to build an image for the child. He can see the equivalence of p.m. times and 24-hour times (such as 8 and 20 coinciding).

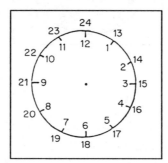

**Figure 14.9**

## Summary for time

The child can progress from reading hours (o'clock) to quarters and halves, to minutes past and minutes to, mastering one stage before he faces the next. The importance of 12 and 60 is stressed, especially the need to start counting again when 12 or 60 is reached. Visual images of clock faces are used to reinforce the calculation procedures.

# Typical Difficulties in Introducing Other Topics

Discussed here are a sample of noteworthy points concerning areas of particular difficulty for dyslexic children.

## Algebra

When a problem quite correctly finishes with a formula, for example $a + b + c$ as the perimeter of the triangle in Figure 14.10, there are children who will be dissatisfied with the lack of a numerical answer. They can usually be convinced by the argument that a formula is an

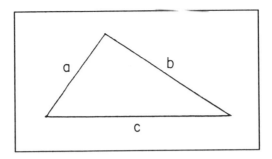

**Figure 14.10**

'instruction' about what to do when the values of $a$, $b$ and $c$ become known. In this sense a formula is superior to a numerical answer, which is only correct for one specific triangle.

Equations are a very important theme, which runs all the way through this subject. The very stylised procedures to be followed for solving them are highly likely to confuse many dyslexics. Therefore, it is necessary to be extremely alert and sensitive, as well as very careful about how this work is presented. At the beginning, the numbers in an equation must be kept simple in order to avoid clouding the main issue. However, children confronted with the equation $x + 3 = 8$ will often rush to give the answer 5 and then be unhappy when their teacher insists (appearing pedantic) that they must set out all the steps properly. Ironically, the very simplicity of the numbers limits their acceptance of the need for a careful procedure. It is necessary to convince children that the need will soon increase and one way is to show them an equation, such as

$$31.2x - x(2.5 - x) = 0.654,$$

which they cannot solve in their heads but may have to solve in later years. This can be followed up by teaching them the motto:

> Look after your equations when they are young, and they will look after you, when you are older.

## Graphs

Mention was made earlier of the value of drawing a graph for some problems. This alternative seems not to occur naturally to dyslexic children. You should therefore lead by example and take every possible opportunity to extract extra information from a problem through the use of a graph. For example, when covering squares and square roots, a curved graph (Figure 14.11) may be plotted for the easy values $x$ and $y$ in Table 14.2.

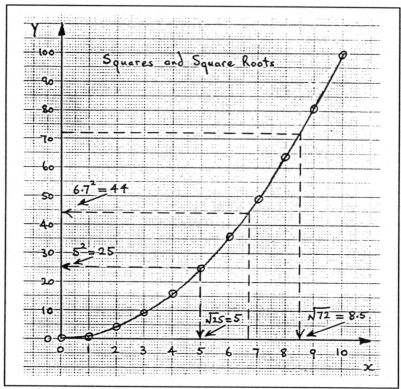

**Figure 14.11**

| Table 14.2 | | | | | | | | | | |
|---|---|---|---|---|---|---|---|---|---|---|
| x | 0 | 1 | 2 | 3 | 4 | 5 | 6 | 7 | 8 | 9 | 10 |
| y | 0 | 1 | 4 | 9 | 16 | 25 | 36 | 49 | 64 | 81 | 100 |

By reading from one scale to the curve, then from the curve to the other scale, the graph can provide much more information than the list of values. Broken lines on the graph show how this is done. Additional information is obtainable in at least two ways:

1. Reading from the $x$ scale to the $y$ scale gives squares, while reading from the $y$ scale to the $x$ scale gives square roots. Through having this dual capability, the graph is providing one of the best ways to demonstrate that squaring and finding square roots are opposite processes, i.e.

$$25 = 5^2$$

so

$$\sqrt{25} = 5.$$

2. Between the 11 plotted points, the curve contains an infinite number of other points, which may be used for values between those in the table. For instance, one of the broken lines shows that $6.7^2 = 44$ to the nearest whole number and another shows that $\sqrt{72} = 8.5$ correct to one decimal place.

## Shape and space

Application of the 'Test of Cognitive Style in Mathematics' (Bath et al., 1986) has indicated that the mathematical style adopted in this branch of the subject, which covers topics like angles, volume and symmetry, is often different from the style for the subject as a whole.

Furthermore, the misconceptions experienced by dyslexics in this branch can produce some of the most confusing mistakes. For example, it has been known for a child to argue long and hard that in the diagram of Figure 14.12: '$y = 40$, because both angles are the same.'

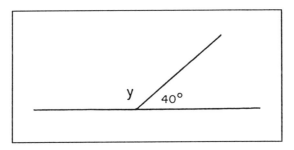

**Figure 14.12**

Discussion showed that the misconception seemed to derive from the observation that both angles were formed with the same pair of straight lines.

# Summary

This chapter's purpose has been to argue the importance to a dyslexic child of the widest possible range of mathematical experiences. Whilst complete coverage of the matter would take another whole book, the chapter includes some examples of when and how to introduce other topics, as well as notes on some of the likely teaching problems.

# Chapter 15
# The Teaching
# Programme at
# Mark College

## Introduction

In this final chapter it is our intention to show how we put our ideas into practice at Mark College in our roles as teachers and organisers in the Mathematics Department. If in many instances we seem to repeat what has been written earlier it is because we regard it as sensible to take our own advice.

We have, however, avoided the repetition of examples at every point and intend this to reduce the amount of text, whilst still making the chapter a useful summary of the whole book.

## Mark College and its Pupils

Mark College is a specialist secondary school for boys who have been diagnosed as dyslexic. Pupils usually join the College at age 11 and leave at age 16. Sixteen pupils of average or above intelligence are admitted each year. Having been diagnosed as dyslexic, it is almost certain that their mathematical achievement does not match their potential. Each pupil must have his learning difficulties dealt with in the context of teaching groups of eight, a size dictated by the need for close individual attention, whilst retaining a sense of community.

Our pupils come from a wide range of backgrounds: social, economic, emotional and educational. In many cases a child will present with considerable anxieties. The elimination of these anxieties is an important priority.

The curriculum is directed towards creating a relaxed, welcoming, empathetic and low-stress atmosphere. When this is achieved, then pupils start to feel confident that they can communicate their difficulties within an environment where their questions are answered empathetically and, rather than just more slowly and more loudly, in alternative ways until an understanding is reached.

The early stages of the course provide work which is easy, in order to restore a sense of success in pupils who may feel (or indeed have been labelled) 'failures'. Equally, the work must not be perceived as too easy or patronising.

New pupils arrive with varying abilities and levels of achievement. In their previous six years of education many will have survived by adopting idiosyncratic methods (or an impressive range of avoidance strategies) and will only have a piecemeal understanding and knowledge of the subject. Our aim is to build on and around what the pupils do understand and know, trying to avoid imposing arbitrary changes which would only add to their confusions. We attempt to provide the structure and organisation which their learning difficulty denies them, while acknowledging that our teaching strategies must enable the full spectrum of learning styles to function (and broaden). Indeed, as we have said earlier, it is our experience that pupils often know more than they realise. They need help with organising and rationalising their information and ideas.

Against this background of intentions, it is critical that we maintain the rigour and integrity of the subject we are teaching. Mathematics is a precise means of communication across the curriculum and in everyday life. In addition, we are obliged to tailor our scheme to the dictates of the National Curriculum through to the appropriate public examinations. However, it is possible to use this programme and work within the constraints to build a sound base for the further studies many of our pupils will pursue.

## The Structure of the Course

The structure is based on a spiral, with a small pitch, so that the child makes frequent returns to the same topics. This provides opportunities for the ever-essential overlearning (and acknowledges the difficulty in achieving mastery of some topics). The spiral rotates around the axis of numeracy. Topics are changed frequently to promote and sustain interest. The topics return quickly and repeatedly so that a pupil's memory meets these important skills and concepts before the work is completely lost. At each return the topic is reviewed and then pushed to a slightly higher level, allowing for progress and giving time for 'digestion' by moving on before the topic is pushed too far.

### Numeracy

The vertical axis of the course begins with:

1.  sorting and classifying;

2.  counting with whole numbers and using them to measure and draw;

3.  adding in whole numbers;

4.  subtracting in whole numbers;

5.  multiplying in whole numbers;

6.  dividing in whole numbers;

7.  understanding about parts of whole numbers;

8.  the four operations for money;

9.  the four operations for decimals;

10. the four operations for fractions.

This axis is regarded as a continuum rather than a collection of separate skills to be acquired independently. The pupil's own characteristic approaches are encouraged. For example, a pupil is liberated (and encouraged) to see a division such as $24 + 4$ as:

- A reverse multiplication, giving 6, because $6 \times 4 = 24$.

- A repeated subtraction down to zero:

    $24 - 4 = 20$     once,         1

    $20 - 4 = 16$     twice,        2

    $16 - 4 = 12$     three times,  3

    $12 - 4 = 8$      four times,   4

    $8 - 4 = 4$       five times,   5

    $4 - 4 = 0$       six times,    6 = answer.

- Repeated additions up to the right answer:

    $0 + 4 = 4$       once,         1

    $4 + 4 = 8$       twice,        2

    etc. to

    $20 + 4 = 24$     six times,    6 = answer.

Note that special attention is given to the number facts for single-figure addition, subtraction (see Chapter 5), multiplication and division (see Chapter 6), since knowing these facts, or having quick and efficient strategies with which to work them out, reduces the load on working/short-term memory during calculations. This knowledge helps both computation and, subsequently, understanding of number.

# General Mathematical Topics

These topics, such as perimeter, area, equations, angle-sums and graphs, are introduced only at the number facility level which the pupil has acquired. The levels of numeracy are carefully organised so that any difficulties are readily identified and easily diagnosed.

The mathematical variety needs to be as wide as possible, as early as possible, in order to maintain motivation and extend experience. In particular, algebra is introduced very early in the form of simple generalisations at the conclusion of a piece of fully understood work. For example, when perimeter has been mastered numerically it is not a large conceptual leap for a child to accept $a + b + c$ as the formula for the perimeter of a triangle. This introduction of algebra also addresses the problem of generalising.

As well as maintaining interest, a wide variety of topics helps to build foundations which are wide, so that difficult areas can be spanned as missing bricks are spanned in a wall. Furthermore, relationships between mathematical topics are revealed and alternative paths are explored and developed.

## Using and applying mathematics

We are committed to the recommendations of the Cockcroft Report (Cockcroft, 1982) and the GCSE requirements for investigations, problem solving and practical work. Thus the Attainment Target 1 of the National Curriculum was also welcomed as supporting this part of our programme. Of the ten 40-minute lessons per week allocated to mathematics, two double lessons are set aside for investigations, problem solving and practical project work. One of these double lessons is likely to involve tasks related to current curriculum work, whilst the content of the other is from a wide range of topics. (Single lessons may be used for shorter tasks.) The pupil's problems with organisation and his need to have experiences on which to build concepts are addressed by these activities. The pupils respond well to such practice and they gain valuable skills for applying their mathematics.

## The use of patterns

We have long advocated the use of patterns in mathematics to act as the mortar which holds the bricks of the subject together (Ashcroft and Chinn, 1992). The importance of patterns was recognised in the 1989 version of the National Curriculum as Attainment Target 5: number/algebra. In our situation we consider patterns and their recognition can:

- streamline the learning of facts;

- add interest and motivation;
- help with conceptual problems;
- rationalise idiosyncrasies;
- provide structure.

### Mental arithmetic

Throughout the course, pupils are encouraged to develop methods of calculating answers in their heads, something most of us do (or try to do) in everyday situations. Whether our expectation is for a correct answer or an estimate, the pupil is encouraged to use mental calculations as his first resort and as his last resort when verifying or checking his answer.

## Classroom Management, Making the Lesson Suit the Pupils

In general, the short attention span and memory deficits of our pupils dictate that a lesson should be divided into short subsections alternating exposition, demonstration, practical work, discussions, practice, etc. The perceptual and organisational difficulties of our pupils dictate the need for clarity of presentation and thorough preparation. Despite the latter requirement, there is a need for a teacher to be flexible enough to change direction in response to problems he may perceive in the course of the lesson.

Board work must be clear and uncluttered, preferably without too much information on display at any one time. The teacher's presentation of work should be both oral and visual. Memory overload must also be avoided.

Teachers should avoid talking (especially about important work) while the pupils are writing. A dyslexic pupil finds it hard enough to copy without this added distraction, which may be further compounded by worrying about what he is not hearing because he is trying to write.

### Spread of ability

Even though the College only admits pupils of average and above intelligence and groups its two mathematics groups according to attainment, there can still be a significant spread of ability and attainment in a class group. So, if the teacher is devoting time to slower pupils, then his organisation and preparation should allow faster pupils to cover selected extra topics so that both faster and slower pupils can progress. There is always a need to see each pupil as an individual. Pupils can also be given the opportunity to help other pupils in order to develop their 'communications level of understanding' (Sharma, 1988).

### Pupils' mathematical cognitive styles

Some pupils follow a rigid, step-by-step, formula/algorithm style when tackling mathematics. This is usually the way this type of learner is best taught. Conversely, other pupils work intuitively and are very answer oriented (see Chapter 2); they may have been stifled and demotivated by being taught in a way which matches the first style and not, therefore, their own style. A good mathematician needs to be flexible and make appropriate use of either style.

Pupils can be helped to find their own best way of working if the teacher:

- begins each lesson with an overall picture of its contents, using both oral and visual stimuli,

- thoroughly explains the logic behind each method,

- offers alternative methods from which to choose,

- puts the work into a familiar context, or relates it to the pupils' own experiences and existing knowledge.

## Evolving Expectations and Emphases

The nature of the pupil's difficulties and his previous experiences in class will often have produced poor levels of achievement and an antipathy for the subject. We begin by trying to restore confidence and build a positive attitude. Success achieved later as the pupil moves up through the College will lead him to recognise his real abilities and raise his expectations to higher levels. We try to equip pupils with enough knowledge and skills to attain their true potential. The mathematics course must allow for development, over a period of five years, between these two extremes. The graph in Figure 15.1 shows how rates of progress are expected to compare with those of 'normal' secondary pupils. The following points are illustrated by the graph:

- Levels of achievement at entry will be lower than 'normal'.

- Initial progress will be slower while confidence is re-established and groundwork is restored.

- At some time in year 9 the progress rate becomes parallel to normal.

- In years 10 and 11 progress needs to be faster than normal if pupils are to reach levels consistent with their intelligence.

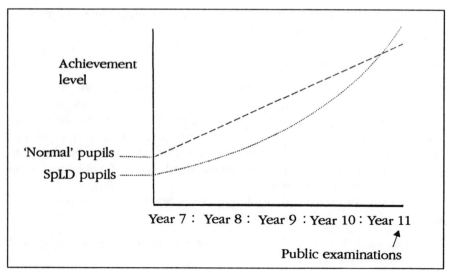

**Figure 15.1**

- Although the progress will be gradual and continuous the developing changes in attitude and motivation require that specific changes in curriculum content and approach are made at the end of year 8 or the beginning of year 9. These different approaches, which allow the curve to be followed and completed, are summarised below.

# Years 7 and 8

In these initial years the course is designed to begin to restore pupils' confidence in their ability to succeed in mathematics. We build on what pupils already know (and often they know more than they realise; it just needs organisation). Much of the work covers the basics in a manner which allows us to:

- revise important work;

- fill in as many gaps as possible;

- rationalise pupils' established ideas which may, at this point, be right, wrong, confused or inefficient;

- by year 9 bring all pupils to a position where their attainment more accurately demonstrates their actual ability.

## Lesson management

Pupils are taught together in groups of (usually) eight. In this situation they gain confidence in their teacher and are encouraged to lose their fear of making mistakes. The size of the group and its ethos enables them to work together, share problems and accept mistakes without stress. The teaching follows a philosophy that is summarised, somewhat simplistically, as 'Mathematics is easy, only writing it down is hard'. The philosophy dictates the following sequence of steps:

1. New topics are introduced via practical work, demonstrations, investigations, discussions and physical experiences. A variety of these is used to facilitate the development and understanding of each concept.

2. An attempt is then made to translate the concept into written form, linking the concrete experiences to the symbolic representation.

3. This leads into worksheets or text-books. The worksheets used at the College start with worked examples, which are related to the earlier experiences. The questions provide practice and revision. The worksheets are the third stage of the procedure and not, therefore, the sole resource for pupils to use for their learning.

### Teaching materials

Pupils in years 7 and 8 use worksheets, as mentioned above, developed by Ashcroft over the past ten years of teaching dyslexics (available from Mark College).

The sheets follow a structured course and are designed to:

- present an advance overview of the section of work to be followed;

- eliminate the need for note-taking, with its inherent risks of slow progress, mistakes, lack of clarity and readability;

- start at the most appropriate point;

- cover only a single topic, so that any point of difficulty can be readily isolated, identified and dealt with;

- contain no more information than can be comfortably digested in one go;

- present work clearly;

- use the fewest possible and simplest words, yet introduce the necessary technical terms carefully;

- incorporate exercises;

- provide a practical revision aid (used as ready-made and organised notes);

- be carefully related to the other sheets.

**Writing paper**

If responses need more space than a worksheet provides, then pupils in years 7 and 8 write on 5 mm squared paper, either in looseleaf form or in exercise books. The squares help with:

- lining up calculations vertically and horizontally;

- setting out tables and charts;

- measurements and diagrams, especially those in centimetres and/or using right angles;

- area problems.

**Calculators**

Since one of the aims of years 7 and 8 is to bring all pupils up to their optimum level of computational competence, the use of calculators is discouraged, except where the work is, for example, repetitive and they are an obvious time saver.

Mental arithmetic is necessary for everyday life and for estimations that check the answers provided by the calculator. Early reliance on a calculator could well delay the acquisition of these mental arithmetic skills.

# Years 9, 10 and 11

During year 9 the pupils' rates of progress are planned to have reached about normal. From this point onwards we see a more internalised positive and motivated attitude.

**Lesson management**

Experience has shown that most pupils have, by now, developed more belief in their ability to succeed in mathematics. Their expectations may also have become quite high. The self-determination to succeed is encouraged by the pupils beginning to work individually for some of their time.

A number of class lessons remain, of course, but individual routes can be provided in lessons. where pupils choose between:

- help or further practice with current work;

- revision of recent or incompletely mastered topics;

- extension work.

It is possible to use published schemes to support this style of structure. We have found good motivation and results with S.M.P. (11–16) Graduated Assessment (School Mathematics Project, 1985–1987).

## Teaching materials

From year 9 pupils are introduced to text-books, that is, they start to use mainstream material. An appropriate book, which becomes familiar and trusted, can provide help and reassurance, especially at examination times. Text-books also provide different viewpoints and a variety in language. The presentation of work in recently published text-books is far more appealing, with good graphics, uncluttered pages and well structured examples. We choose our text-books carefully, so as not to lose the changes in attitude we have worked so hard to achieve.

We have had success with the text-books listed in the Appendix.

## Writing paper

During year 10, or earlier if they so choose, pupils change from 5 mm squared paper to 8 mm lined paper. Thus, we become aligned with practice in 'normal' schools and ready for examinations where lined paper is provided.

## Calculators

In years 9, 10 and 11 the use of calculators becomes increasingly obligatory. Indeed, their use is expected at GCSE. We recommend the use of a simple solar-powered calculator with scientific functions, including fractions, percentage, degrees/minutes/seconds, and one which will not resort to scientific form for all answers. A good machine can be bought cheaply. Calculators are an ideal aid for short-term memory and can help compensate for the pupils' remaining computational difficulties (which tend to be a matter of speed). We attempt to filter out logic and keying errors by encouraging methods of checking (usually estimates made mentally). The introduction and use of specific calculator functions are carried out mainly on the basis of need, as with the trigonometric functions for example. Lessons can, however, be set aside for the exploration of other functions such as $n!$ (factorial $n$), which are of investigational rather than curricular interest.

# Public Examinations

Success in public examinations is in no way inconsistent with the objectives of the curriculum, although early work and progress may make it look that way. Rather, success in these examinations is the yard-stick against which pupils will be measured when they leave and a challenge they are ready to face. Results at GCSE are achievable for all our pupils according to their abilities and motivation.

We regard it as our responsibility to use the system as efficiently and effectively as possible and to apply for whatever special provisions are available for each pupil on an individual basis. (Most usually this is 25% extra time and sometimes a reader or amanuensis.)

In the near future testing will be carried out as part of the National Curriculum. Testing for our age range will be at Key Stage 3 and Key Stage 4 (this latter testing will replace GCSE). Testing at Key Stage 3 will occur in year 9. The graph given in Figure 15.1 suggests this is the year when our pupils are typically the furthest behind 'normal' pupils. Despite this potential disadvantage, we prefer to maintain the integrity of our five-year programme, rather than pursue the counter-productive course of pushing our pupils too early for this stage. Our main examination target, therefore, is success at Key Stage 4.

The system for GCSE mathematics examinations has always placed great responsibility on schools for entering pupils at the correct level. This responsibility seems (on present information) more likely to increase rather than decrease when Key Stage 4 testing replaces GCSE in 1994. This will require us to refine decisions about levels of entry continuously over years 9, 10 and 11. The unpredictable effects of emotional pressure on dyslexics at examination time makes taking these decisions a very difficult (and arguably avoidable) task.

At Mark College we carefully monitor progress throughout the year and through the levels of the National Curriculum, measuring against the separate Attainment Targets. A pupil's progress, as monitored in class combined with results from tests and College examinations, is used to place him in the teaching group that is most suitable for his current learning needs and long-term potential. If this system remains effective then, when public examinations arrive, decisions about levels of entry virtually make themselves.

## Assessment

Pupils are assessed regularly for the purpose of:

- placement in appropriate teaching groups;

- diagnosis of difficulties;

- monitoring progress;

- distinguishing mathematical cognitive style.

We make it clear to the pupils, most of whom have a long history of 'being tested', that our test results are for internal consumption only. This reduces their fear of the testing process to a level where it should only be distasteful!

## Placement in teaching groups

Although our intake is of average or above-average intelligence, the pupils have a wide range of difficulties, which produce a full spectrum of mathematical achievements and abilities. We regard it as important to group pupils according to their current attainment level. In this arrangement the diversity of their learning difficulties is not further compounded by great divides of ability. Pupils seem to feel safest and are more comfortable when asking questions or airing their problems if they are among those with similar levels of difficulty and achievement. There is flexibility of movement between groups as pupils move towards their full potential and particularly as public examinations approach.

## Monitoring progress

Many standardised tests lead to a 'mathematical' age or quotient. This single figure is used to represent the pupil's current level of achievement, which can then be compared to previous figures as one way to monitor progress. These tests are given at the same or similar times each year. We treat test results with caution (see Chapter 3) and always consider them in conjunction with progress in class, and with changes over a variety of situations, to obtain a real measure of progress.

We use the following standardised tests (which are published by Hodder and Stoughton): Basic Number Screening Test (Gillham and Hesse, 1987); Graded Arithmetic – Mathematics Test, Junior and Senior Levels (Vernon and Miller, 1986).

To assess mathematical learning/cognitive style, we use the Test of Cognitive Style in Mathematics (Bath et al., 1986). It is used to distinguish between the step-by-step inchworm and the intuitive, holistic grasshopper. This American test is for use with individual pupils and provides a measure of the pupil's position on the continuum of styles from extreme inchworm to extreme grasshopper.

## Diagnosis of difficulties

Some standardised tests are designed to test mathematical subskills separately so that particular problem areas can be identified. The results of these types of test can be used to direct subsequent teaching towards specific areas of weakness. An example of such a test is 'The Profile of Mathematical Skills' (France, 1976).

For times-table and basic-addition facts testing we test twice, once at five-second intervals to test immediate recall and once at 15-second intervals to allow pupils to utilise strategies.

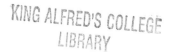

**The Mark College test**

The College has its own test designed for dyslexic mathematicians (see Appendix 3). The test, written by Ashcroft, is based on a survey of the errors most commonly made by dyslexics (Joffe, 1980). It consists of items based on the areas where these errors occur. Consequently it helps with the diagnostic process and in measuring the effectiveness of remediation.

**Schedule of assessment**

To gain an overview of the levels of achievement and rates of progress of both groups and individuals, various standardised tests are applied at fixed points in the five-year College academic cycle. These are detailed in Table 15.1.

**Table 15.1.** Application of Standard Tests

| Year group<br>Approx. age | 7<br>11–12 | | 8<br>12–13 | | 9<br>13–14 | | 10<br>14–15 | | 11<br>15–16 | |
|---|---|---|---|---|---|---|---|---|---|---|
| When applied | Sep. | Mar. | Sep. | Mar. | Sep. | Mar. | Sep. | Mar. | Sep. | Mar. |
| Mark College Test – Ashcroft | ✳ | | ✳ | | | | | | | |
| Basic Number Screening Test – Gillham and Hesse | ✳ | ✳ | ✳ | ✳ | ✳ | | | | | |
| Profile of Mathematical Skills – France | | | | | ✳ | | | | | |
| Graded Arithmetic – Mathematics Test | | | | | | | | | | |
| (i) Junior Level | | | | ✳ | ✳ | ✳ | | | | |
| (ii) Senior Level – Vernon and Miller | | | | | | ✳ | ✳ | ✳ | ✳ | ✳ |

**In-house examinations**

The pupils take a College examination twice a year. This helps to prepare them for the rigours of public examinations and encourages revision and study skills. We give two papers each time:

- Paper 1 consists of short questions and tests the width of pupils' knowledge and their accuracy.

- Paper 2 consists of longer questions and tests the depth of pupils' understanding and their problem-solving abilities.

### The National Curriculum

We have always adapted our work towards the National Curriculum, though the frequency of changes in the Curriculum is not as easy to keep up with as we would sometimes like. We had anticipated the need to split the work into five Attainment Target areas and appreciate the structure inherent in the programme, which is so helpful to our pupils.

Our course for years 7 and 8 requires that pupils are taught at levels below those required at Key Stage 3 (which looks to teaching over levels 3 to 8) for part of the time. It would be very counter-productive to begin all our introductory work at level 3. The NCC 'Non-Statutory Guidance' (1989) allows that 'certain pupils will benefit from work at a lower level in order to help them to consolidate a particular skill'.

In essence, then, we have parity at Key Stage 4 as our ultimate goal, but the nature of our pupils and the programme we have designed to address their needs means that we may not be on target (as defined by the National Curriculum) at earlier stages.

## Summary

We have covered all the contributing factors which influenced the design of our programme. The intention was to guide rather than dictate, as other situations may require different responses to factors other than the ones we have chosen.

# Appendices

# Appendix 1: Books, Journals, Tests and Games

## Books

The following list collects some useful titles together (and provides ISBN details). Note that the books, together with those cited in the text of the book, are given, in alphabetical order, in the *References* section.

### Background

Copeland, R.W. (1984). *How Children Learn Mathematics: Teaching Implications of Piaget's Research.* New York: Macmillan. 0-02-324770-3

Crawley, J.F. (1985). *Cognitive Strategies and Mathematics for the Learning Disabled.* Rockville, MD: Aspen Systems Corporation. 0-87189-120-4

Ernst, P. (ed.) (1989). *Mathematics Teaching: The State of the Art.* Lewes: Falmer Press. 1-85000-461-7 (pbk)

Krutetskii, V.A. (1976). *The Psychology of Mathematical Abilities in School-children.* Chicago: University of Chicago Press. 0220-45492-4

Miles, T.R. and Miles, E. (eds) (1992). *Dyslexia and Mathematics.* London: Routledge. 0-415-04987-3 (pbk)

Skemp, R.R. (1986). *The Psychology of Learning Mathematics,* 2nd edition. Harmondsworth: Pelican. 0-14-022668-0

Stoltz, C. and Brown, M. (1982). *Low Attainers in Mathematics 5-16.* School Council Publications. London: Methuen. 0-423-51020-7

### Teaching

Ashlock, R.B. (1982). *Error Patterns in Computation.* Columbus, OH: Charles E. Merrill. 0-675-09880-7

Ashlock, R., Johnson, M., Wilson, J. and Jones, W. (1983). *Guiding Each Child's Learning of Mathematics.* Columbus, OH: Charles E. Merrill. 0-675-20023-7

Bley, N. and Thornton, C. (1989). *Teaching Mathematics to the Learning Disabled.* Pro-Ed (8700 Shoal Creek Boulevard, Austin, TX 78758-9965). 0-89079-200-3

Burge, V. (1986). *Basic Numeracy.* Farnham: Helen Arkell Centre. 0-9506070-6-1

Deboys, M. and Pitt, E. (1988). *Lines of Development in Primary Mathematics,* 3rd edition. Belfast: Blackstaff Press. 0-85640-194-3

Geere, B. (undated). *Seven Ways to Help Your Child with Maths.* Seven Ways Series, published by Barbara Geere

Henderson, A. (1989). *Maths and Dyslexics.* St David's College, Llandudno. 0-9512529-1-7

Reisman, F. (1978). *A Guide to the Diagnostic Teaching of Arithmetic,* 2nd edition. Columbus, OH: Charles E. Merrill. 0-675-008397-4

## Journals

*Focus on Learning Problems in Mathematics.* Center for Teaching/Learning of Mathematics, P.O. Box 3149, Framingham, MA 01701, USA.

*Math Notebook.* Center for Teaching/Learning of Mathematics, P.O. Box 3149, Framingham, MA 01701, USA.

## Videos

*The Teaching and Learning of Mathematics.* Mahesh Sharma. Produced by Oxford Polytechnic (now Oxford Brookes University). Available from Mrs P. Brazil, The Warren, Mapledurham, Reading RG4 7TQ.

## Tests

*Basic Number Screening Test* (1987). Gillham, W. and Hesse, K. Sevenoaks: Hodder and Stoughton.

*Graded Arithmetic – Mathematics Test* (1986). Vernon, P. with the assistance of Miller, K. Sevenoaks: Hodder and Stoughton.

*Mathematics Learning Style Inventory* (1993). Chinn, S.J. and Bath, J.B. Belford, Northumberland: Ann Arbor (UK only). To be published.

*Profile of Mathematics Skills* (1979). France, N. Windsor: NFER-Nelson.

*Test of Cognitive Style in Mathematics* (1986). Bath, J.B., Chinn, S.J. and Knox, D.E. East Aurora, NY: Slosson.

*Test of Early Mathematics Ability* (2nd edition) (1990). Ginsburg, H.P. and Baroody, A.J. Pro-Ed (8700 Shoal Creek Boulevard, Austin, TX 78758-9965).

Wide Range Achievement Test (revised edition) (1984). Jastak, S.J. and Jastak, G.S. Jastak Associates, Inc. (15 Ashley Place, Suite 1A, Wilmington, DE 19804).

*Mathematics 8–12* (1984). National Foundation for Educational Research with Brighouse, A., Godber, D. and Patilla, P. Windsor: NFER-Nelson.

## Games and activities

Bolt, B. (1982). *Mathematical Activities. A Resource Book for Teachers.* Cambridge University Press. 0-521-28518-6. (Also, *More Mathematical Activities; Even More Mathematical Activities; The Amazing Mathematical Amusement Arcade.*)

Burton, L. (1984). *Thinking Things Through. Problem Solving in Mathematics.* Oxford: Blackwell. 0-631-13813-7

Kirkby, D. has written several books featuring games and activities, including:

*Starting Games* (1993). Glasgow: Collins Educational. 0-00312-5548

*More Games* (1993). Glasgow: Collins Educational. 0-00312-5556

*Go Further with Games* (1989). London: Unwin Hyman. 0-0444-8099-7

*Games in the Teaching of Mathematics* (1992). Cambridge: Cambridge University Press. 0-521-42320-1

Mottershead, L. (1978). *Sources of Mathematical Discovery.* Oxford: Blackwell. 0-631-10221-3

# Appendix 2: Teaching Materials

Some materials can be made, others have to be bought. Unless a supplier is specified, the material is widely available from educational suppliers such as Hope, NES, etc. (see addresses below).

Dominoes
Playing cards
Blank playing cards
Money (plastic or real)
Base ten blocks ( from NES, Hope or Taskmaster)
Poker chips (import 'real' ones from America)
Large (2 cm+) counters
Cocktail sticks (in boxes of 100, bundles of 10 and singly)
Squared paper
Place value cards (make your own)
Abacus
Geo boards
Dice (various shapes and values; blank six-sided dice are obtainable)
Cuisenaire rods (from Cuisenaire Company)
Film tubs from 35 mm film
Multi-link cubes
Uni-fix cubes
Metre rules: mm divisions, cm divisions and dm divisions
Pipe cleaners
Number square, 1 to 100, with counters
Clock faces (synchronised hands)
Calculators
Pie chart scales
10 dm cube (1 litre)
Tape measure
Trundle wheel
Kitchen scales

## Suppliers' addresses

Cuisenaire Company, 11 Crown Street, Reading, RG1 2TQ.
Galt Educational, Cheadle, Cheshire, SK8 2PN.
Hope Education Ltd, Orb Mill, Huddersfield Road, Waterhead, Oldham, Lancs, OL4 2ST.
NES, Ludlow Hill Road, West Bridgford, Notts, NG2 6HD.
Philip and Tacey, North Way, Andover, Hampshire, SP10 5BA.
Taskmaster Ltd, Morris Street, Leicester, LE2 6BR.

# Appendix 3: The Ashcroft Maths Test

**Name:**_____     **Date:**_____

(1)
$$
\begin{array}{r}
39 \\
+\,45 \\
\hline
\end{array}
$$

(2)
$$
\begin{array}{r}
72 \\
-5 \\
\hline
\end{array}
$$

(3)
$$
\begin{array}{r}
734 \\
-261 \\
\hline
\end{array}
$$

(4)
$$
\begin{array}{r}
47 \\
\times\,3 \\
\hline
\end{array}
$$

(5)   $2\overline{)806}$

(6)   $3\overline{)222}$

(7)
$$
\begin{array}{r}
3.41 \\
\times\,.2 \\
\hline
\end{array}
$$

(8)   $6.39 + .3$

$\overline{)\phantom{xxx}}$

*Write your answers to questions (9) to (14) on the lines at the side.*

(9)    Write in figures

    (a)   Three Hundred and Forty Seven          _____

    (b)   Five Pounds Two pence          _____

(10)   What value has the 8 in

    (a)   836          _____

    (b)   285          _____

(11)     $3.6 + 23 + 7 + 2.54 + 864$

(Use the space below for your working)

_____

(12)     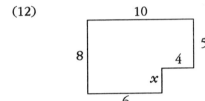                                    (Not to scale)

How long is the side marked *x*?                _____

(13)     Find the sum of 5 and 3                        _____

(14)     Subtract 2 from 7                                 _____

*For problems (15) to (18), decide which operation you would do to find the answer.*

*Choose from*          Add          +

                       Subtract     —

                       Multiply     ×

                       Divide       +

*Put one **sign** in each box*                          Operation

(15)    David is 13 years old and his brother
        James is two years younger.               13 ☐ 2
        How old is James?


(16)    A classroom has 5 rows of chairs, with
        3 chairs in each row.                       5 ☐ 3
        How many chairs are there altogether?


(17)    4 boys pay 80p altogether to take a bus
        ride.                                       80 ☐ 4
        How much does each boy pay?


(18)    There are 7 girls in a room. How many
        will there be if 4 more come in?             7 ☐ 4

# References

ASHCROFT, J.R. and CHINN, S.J. (1992). In Miles, T.R. and Miles, E. (eds). *Dyslexia and Mathematics*, p. 23. Routledge. London.

ASHLOCK, R., JOHNSON, M., WILSON, J. and JONES, W. (1983). *Guiding Each Child's Learning of Mathematics*. Columbus, OH: Merrill.

ASHLOCK, R.B. (1982). *Error Patterns in Computation*. Columbus, OH: Merrill.

AUSTIN, J.D.,(1982). Children with a Learning Disability in Mathematics. *School Science and Mathematics*, 201–208.

BATH, J.B., CHINN, S.J. and KNOX, D.E. (1986). *The Test of Cognitive Style in Mathematics*. East Aurora, NY: Slosson.

BATH, J.B. and KNOX, D.E. (1984). Two styles of performing mathematics. In Bath, J.B., Chinn, S.J. and Knox, D.E. (Eds), *Dyslexia: Research and its Application to the Adolescent*. Bath: Better Books.

BLEY, N. and THORNTON, C. (1989). *Teaching Mathematics to the Learning Disabled*. Pro-Ed (8700 Shoal Creek Boulevard, Austin, TX 78758-9965).

BOLT, B. (1982). *Mathematical Activities. A Resource Book for Teachers*. Cambridge: Cambridge University Press.

BOLT, B. (1982). *More Mathematical Activities*. Cambridge: Cambridge University Press.

BOLT, B. (1983). *Even More Mathematical Activities*. Cambridge: Cambridge University Press.

BOLT, B. (1984). *The Amazing Mathematical Amusement Arcade*. Cambridge: Cambridge University Press.

BURGE, V. (1986). *Basic Numeracy*. Farnham: Helen Arkell Centre.

BURTON, L. (1984). *Thinking Things Through. Problem Solving in Mathematics*. Oxford: Blackwell.

BUXTON, L. (1981). *Do You Panic About Maths?* London: Heinemann.

CHASTY, H.T. (1989). The challenge of specific learning difficulties. *Proceedings of the First International Conference of the British Dyslexia Association*. Reading: BDA.

CHINN, S.J. (1991). Factors to consider when designing a test protocol in mathematics for dyslexics. In Snowling, M. and Thomson, M. (Eds), *Dyslexia: Integrating Theory and Practice*. London: Whurr.

CHINN, S.J. (1992). Individual diagnosis and cognitive style. In Miles, T.R. and Miles, E. (Eds), *Dyslexia and Mathematics*. London: Routledge.

CHINN, S.J. and BATH, J.B. (1993). *Mathematics Learning Style Inventory*. Belford, Northumberland: Ann Arbor. To be published.

221

COBB, P. (1991). Reconstructing elementary school mathematics. *Focus on Learning Problems in Mathematics*, **13** (2), 3–32.

COCKCROFT, W.H. (1982). *Mathematics Counts*. London: HMSO.

COPE, C.L. (1988). Math anxiety and math avoidance in college freshmen. *Focus on Learning Problems in Mathematics*, **10** (1), 1–13.

COPELAND, R.W. (1984). *How Children Learn Mathematics. Teaching Implications of Piaget's Research*. New York: Macmillan.

CRAWLEY, J.F. (1985). *Cognitive Strategies and Mathematics for the Learning Disabled*. Rockville, MD: Aspen Systems Corporation.

CRITCHLEY, McD. (1970). The neurological approach in assessment and teaching of dyslexic children. In White, F.A. and Naidoo, S. (Eds), *Assessment and Teaching of Dyslexic Children*. London: ICAA.

DE BONO, E. (1970). *Lateral Thinking: A Textbook of Creativity*. London: Ward Lock Educational.

DEBOYS, M. and PITT, E. (1988). *Lines of Development in Primary Mathematics*, 3rd edition. Belfast: Blackstaff Press.

DUFFIN, J. (1991). Oh yes you can! *Times Educational Supplement*, 10 May, p.49.

ERNST, P. (Ed.). (1989). *Mathematics Teaching: The State of the Art*. Lewes: Falmer Press.

FRANCE, N. (1979). *The Profile of Mathematical Skills*. Windsor: NFER-Nelson.

GEERE, B. (undated). *Seven Ways to Help Your Child with Maths*. Seven Ways Series, published by Barbara Geere.

GILLHAM, W. and HESSE, K. (1987). *Basic Number Screening Test*. Sevenoaks: Hodder and Stoughton.

GINSBURG, H.P. and BAROODY, A.J. (1990). *Test of Early Mathematics Ability*, 2nd edition. Pro-Ed (8700 Shoal Creek Boulevard, Austin, TX 78758-9965).

HART, K. (1978). *Children's Understanding of Mathematics: 11–16*. London: John Murray.

HART, K. (1989). There is little connection. In Ernst, P. (Ed.), *Mathematics Teaching: The State of the Art*. Lewes: Falmer Press.

HARVEY, R. (1982). "I can keep going up if I want to": One Way of Looking at learning mathematics. In Harvey, R., Kerslake, D., Shuard, H, and Torbe, M. (Eds), *Language Teaching and Learning. 6. Mathematics*. London: Ward Lock Educational.

HENDERSON, A. (1989). *Maths and Dyslexics*. Llandudno: St David's College.

HOMAN, D.R. (1970). The child with a learning disability in arithmetic. *The Arithmetic Teacher*, **18**, 199–203

JASTAK, S.J. and JASTAK, G.S. (1984). *Wide Range Achievement Test*, revised edition. Jastak Associates, Inc. (15 Ashley Place, Suite 1A, Wilmington, DE 19804).

JOFFE, L. (1980). Dyslexia and attainment in school mathematics: Part 2, Error types and remediation. *Dyslexia Review*, **3** (2), 12–18.

JOFFE, L. (1983). School mathematics and dyslexia...a matter of verbal labelling, generalisation, horses and carts. *Cambridge Journal of Education*, **13** (3), 22–27.

KANE, N. and KANE, M. (1979). Comparison of right and left hemisphere functions. *The Gifted Child Quarterly*, **23** (1), 157–167.

KAVANAGH, J.K. and TRUSS, T.J. (Eds) (1988). *Learning Disabilities: Proceedings of the National Conference*. Parkton, MD: York Press.

KENNEDY, L.M. (1975). *Guiding Children to Mathematical Discovery*. Belmont, CA: Wadsworth.

KIBEL, M. (1992). Linking language to action. In Miles, T.R. and Miles, E. (Eds), *Dyslexia and Mathematics*. London: Routledge.

KIRKBY, D. (1989). *Go Further with Games*. London: Unwin Hyman.

KIRKBY, D. (1992). *Games in the Teaching of Mathematics*. Cambridge University Press.

KIRKBY, D. (1993). *Starting Games*. Glasgow: Collins Educational.

KIRKBY, D. (1993). *More Games*. Glasgow: Collins Educational.

KRUTETSKII, V.A. (1976). In Kilpatric, J. and Wirszup I. (Eds), *The Psychology of Mathematical Abilities in School Children*. Chicago: University of Chicago Press.

KUBRICK, S. and RUDNICK, J.A. (1980). *Problem Solving – A Handbook for Teachers*. Needham Heights, NY: Allyn and Bacon.

LANE, C. (1992). Now listen hear. *Special Children*, **54**, 12–14.

LANE, C. and CHINN, S.J. (1986). Learning by self-voice echo. *Academic Therapy*, **21**, 477–481.

LLEWELLYN, S. and GREER, A. (1983). *Mathematics the Basic Skills*. Cheltenham: Stanley Thornes.

LUCHINS, A.S. (1942). Mechanisation in problem solving: the effect of Einstellung. *Psychological Monographs*, **54** (6).

McDOUGAL, S. (1990). *Table Time. The Exciting New Way to Learn Multiplication Tables*. Bromley: Harrap.

McLEISH, J. (1991). *Number*. London: Bloomsbury.

MILES, E. (1992). Reading and writing in mathematics. In Miles, T.R. and Miles, E. (Eds), *Dyslexia and Mathematics*. London: Routledge.

MILES, T.R. (1983). *Dyslexia: The Pattern of Difficulties*. Oxford: Blackwell.

MILES, T.R. (1993). *Dyslexia: The Pattern of Difficulties*, 2nd edition. London: Whurr.

MILES, T.R. and MILES, E. (Eds) (1992). *Dyslexia and Mathematics*. London: Routledge.

MOTTERSHEAD, L. (1978). *Sources of Mathematical Discovery*. Oxford: Blackwell.

NATIONAL CURRICULUM COUNCIL (1989). The order of activities should be flexible. *Mathematics Non-Statutory Guidance*, §5.3, p. B.8.

NATIONAL FOUNDATION FOR EDUCATIONAL RESEARCH with BRIGHOUSE, A., GODBER, D. and PATILLA, P. (1984). *Mathematics 8–12*. Windsor: NFER-Nelson.

POLYA, G. (1962). *Mathematical Discovery*, Vol. 1. New York: Wiley.

PRITCHARD, R.A., MILES, T.R., CHINN, S.J. and TAGGART, A.T. (1989). Dyslexia and knowledge of number facts. *Links*, **14** (3), 17–20.

PUMPHREY, P.D. and REASON, R. (1991). *Specific Learning Difficulties (Dyslexia): Challenges and Responses*. Windsor: NFER-Nelson.

RAYNER, D. (1987). *Mathematics for GCSE*, Books 1 and 2. Oxford: Oxford University Press.

RAYNER, D. (1988). *General Mathematics: Revision and Practice*. Oxford: Oxford University Press.

REISMAN, F. (1978). *A Guide to the Diagnostic Teaching of Arithmetic*, 2nd edition. Columbus, OH: Charles E. Merrill.

SCHOOL MATHEMATICS PROJECT (1985–1987). S.M.P. *(11–16)*. *Green Series*. Cambridge: Cambridge University Press.

SHARMA, M.C. (1986). Dyscalculia and other learning problems in arithmetic: a historical prospective. *Focus on Learning Problems in Mathematics*, **8** (3,4), 7–45.

SHARMA, M.C. (1988). Levels of knowing mathematics. *Math Notebook*, **6** (1,2).

SHARMA, M.C. (1988). Mathematics workshop at Mark College.

SHARMA, M.C. (1989). Mathematics learning personality. *Math Notebook*, **7** (1,2).

SKEMP, R.R. (1981). *The Psychology of Learning Mathematics*. Harmondsworth: Penguin.

SKEMP, R.R. (1986). *The Psychology of Learning Mathematics*, 2nd edition. Harmondsworth: Pelican.

STEEVES, J. (1979). Multisensory math: an instructional approach to help the LD child. *Focus on Learning Problems in Mathematics*, 1 (2), 51-62.

STOLTZ, C. and BROWN, M. (1982). *Low Attainers in Mathematics 5-16*. School Council Publications. London: Methuen.

SUTHERLAND, P. (1988). Dyscalculia. Sum cause for concern? *Times Educational Supplement*, 18 March 1988.

VERNON, P. with the assistance of MILLER, K. (1986). *Graded Arithmetic – Mathematics Test*. Sevenoaks: Hodder and Stoughton.

WHEATLEY, G.H. (1977). The right hemisphere's role in problem solving. *The Arithmetic Teacher*, 25, 36-39.

WHEATLEY, G.H., FRANKLAND, R.L., MITCHELL, O.R. and KRAFT, R. (1978). Hemispheric specialization and cognitive development: implications for mathematics education. *Journal for Research in Mathematics Education*, 9, 20-32.

WILSON, J. and SADOWSKI, B. (Eds) (1976). *The Maryland Diagnostic Test and Interview Protocols*. Arithmetic Center, University of Maryland.

# Index